ALSO BY YVONNE F. CONTE

Serious Laughter
Live a happier, healthier, more productive life!

Bits of Joy
150 ideas that will make you jump for joy.

Frankie Wonders, "What Happened Today?"
A look at September 11 through the eyes of a child.

Remarkable Women of Faith
In-depth testimonies from some of America's
most remarkable women of faith.
co-authored by Yvonne Conte, Ann Jillian, and Jennifer O'Neil

Make a Big Deal
How to be a motivational speaker
and bestselling author.

D0167883

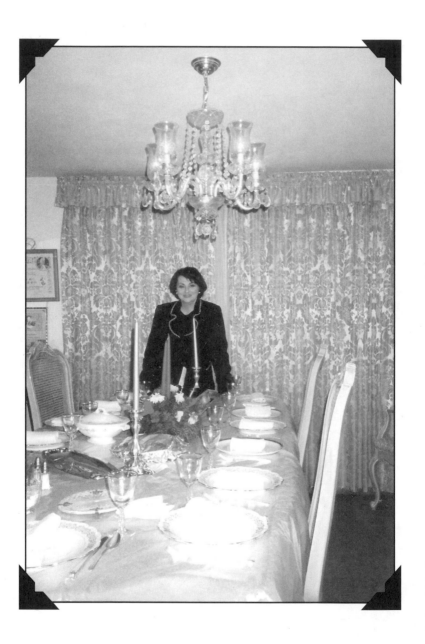

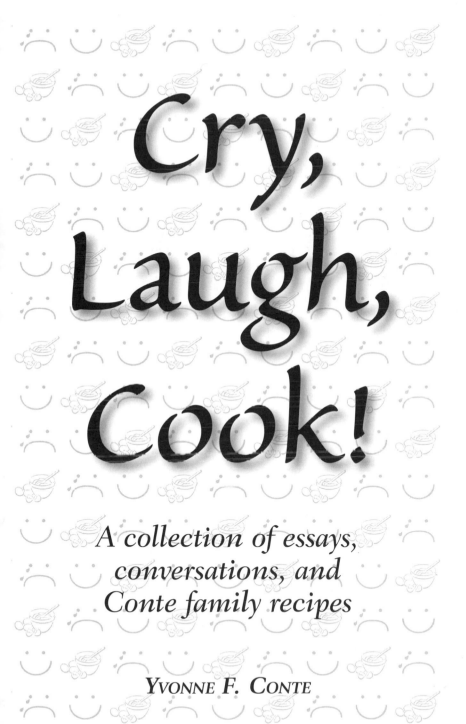

Cry, Laugh, Cook!

A collection of essays, conversations, and Conte family recipes

YVONNE F. CONTE

Cry, Laugh, Cook!
A collection of essays, conversations, and Conte family recipes.
by Yvonne F. Conte

Published by Amsterdam Berwick Publishing

Design and Typesetting by Richard Groff/TypeSmith

Ordering information—Individual Sales: All Amsterdam-Berwick books are available through most bookstores. They may also be ordered on line at: www.yvonneconte.com and www.amazon.com. Quantity Discounts: Purchases used as college textbooks and/or client gifts may qualify for special discounts and are available to bulk purchasers by contacting:
Special Sales Department
Amsterdam Berwick Publishing
4736 Onondaga Blvd. Suite 231
Syracuse, NY 13219
315.487.3771

Printed in the United States of America

10 9 8 7 6 5 4 3 2 1

First Edition

Library of Congress Cataloging-in-Publication Data
Conte, Yvonne F., 1951–
    Cry, laugh, cook! : A collection of essays, conversations, and Conte family recipes / Yvonne F. Conte—Amsterdam Berwick Publishing.
        p.   cm.
    1. Self-realization.   2. American wit and humor.   3. Cooking.
I. Title.

ISBN 978-0-9665336-7-5

For
Barbara Martin Holbrook
and
Theresa Pilato Zbick

We have cried together,
laughed together,
and cooked together,
because that's what true friends do.

"I am leaving you with a gift—peace of mind and heart."

John 14:27

"Breathe it in my friends and know that you have
the gift of peace whenever you want it."

Vonnie

Contents

Foreword

How often do we talk about our lives growing up? Do we think about how our relationships with our siblings have changed over the years? Do we recognize the humor all around us? What lessons have we learned, what traits do we embrace, and what foods take us back home? This is the fabric of our lives—our history. Recording the experiences and ideals that carry us through life is one of the greatest gifts we can give to our family. This book is an example of one way to share the gift of who we are.

The book will not be read just once. The threads of family life are vivid and compelling. The conversations are a reminder of the importance of humor in everyday life. And the recipes are simply delicious home cooking. We may think the book will find a place on the bookshelf, but it will be more at home in the kitchen.

So here is the simple recipe:

Read about a vibrant life, find the humor in everyday living, and complete the cycle by sitting down with those close to you for a wonderful, home-cooked meal.

Enjoy!

Carla Jonquil

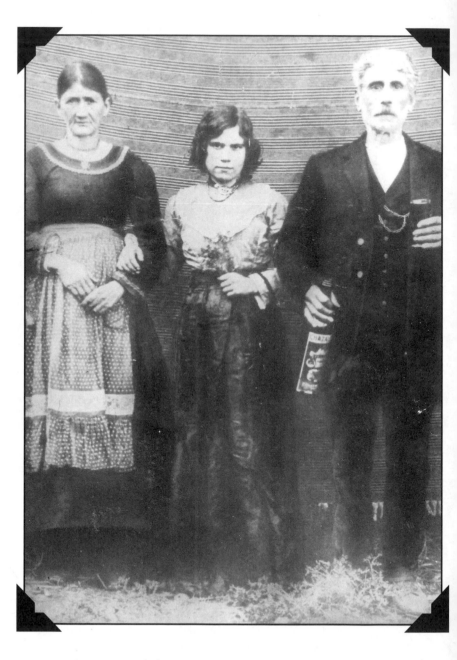

Francesca DiVito Conte, Maria Conte, Francesco Conte
Amaroni, Italy

Introduction

The Conte Family traces our origin to Amaroni, a small town in the Province of Catanzaro, in southern Italy, in the Region of Calabria. My great grandparents, Francesco and Francesca (DiVito) Conte had three sons and two daughters. Their eldest son was my grandfather, Antonio Conte. We called him Pa. He came to this country as a young boy and hoped for a good life in the new world. He married Philomena Marrotta and had four children. The eldest was my father, Frances William Conte. My dad came from a strong, dedicated, and loyal family. He knew the power of that kind of family strength and he passed that knowledge down to my sisters and me. Somehow that made me feel very safe and protected as a child growing up in the '50s and '60s. I always knew my family had my back, no matter what. They would always be there for me; I could count on that. If ever there was a disagreement with one of us kids, Dad would look at us and say, "That's your sister. You're family. I don't want to hear anymore. Kiss and make up." And we always did. My father would not tolerate any sort of discord. We *cried* a little bit, we *laughed* a little bit, and then Daddy would get us in the kitchen and we'd *cook!*

Somehow a wonderful meal and sitting around the table together made everything all right. He taught me that nothing is as important as the family. He has been gone now since 1995 and much has changed. Our families have gotten bigger and some of our traditions have gone by the wayside. I think that happens in most families as time goes on.

I wrote this book because I want my grandchildren to know that same kind of family strength and loyalty that I grew up with. I think it's time for Americans to go back to their roots and back to the values, respect, and beliefs that this country was founded on.

In the first section you will find a collection of essays. Some are funny, some are emotional, and some are just my random thoughts. I've tried to be descriptive so that you can almost hear the laughter from my many Conte, Gerace, Scarano, and Paone cousins, smell the aromas, and envision us around the table.

The second section offers the same kind of values, respect, and beliefs in conversations with Gary Dunes, a long-time fixture in the Central New York radio market. The third section is my real gift to you: I'm giving away all the family secrets! Recipes from three generations of Contes fill the pages. I'm telling you, you can almost smell the sauce. I hope you enjoy this book. Of everything I've ever written, this book offers more of me—my heart and soul, my thoughts and dreams, and the food that made me who I am. Mmmm, *molto bene!* Enjoy!

Yvonne

"My task, which I am trying to achieve by the power of the written word, to make you hear, to make you feel—it is, before all, to make you see. That and no more, and it is everything."
Joseph Conrad

Acknowledgments

Thank You!

Dawn Christensen at Loretta LaRoche and Company and The Humor Potential for having faith in my talents and sending me out to speak to some of the best companies and groups in the country.

Judy Kelly and Gary Dunes at WSEN 92.1 FM for taking a chance and generously allowing this little Italian girl to have a voice every week on the radio.

NBC3 (Syracuse) News Anchor Laura Hand for first bringing my message to the masses on the Noon News. You have been a great friend and mentor. You have no idea how that helped Humor Advantage, Inc., to grow.

Ryan Prucker and everyone at Image Light Marketing for believing so passionately in my worth. Your enthusiasm and energy is contagious. Thanks for going to the mountaintop and shouting out my name.

Tod Baker at Thomson Shore Printing and Richard Groff at TypeSmith for your patience and kindness and for allowing me to change my mind.

To the kindest person I know: Carla Conte Jonquil. You always say yes and you always bring homemade baked goods.

Terri Zbick—without your encouragement and love this book would never have come together. Thank you for your confidence in me and for pushing me to "put my stories in a book."

John and Gwen Elmer and my family at the Syracuse Vineyard for spiritual guidance and mentoring, for helping me to grow in Christ and showing me honest Christian love. A special thanks to Lisa Andrews and Sheila DeRose for helping me to grow, for listening, and for your constant and beautiful friendship.

Barbara Holbrook, who always says things that make me laugh, like "The bigger the hair, the closer to God." Thank you for our daily long-distance chats, for loving me unconditionally, for helping me see that every setback is just a setup for a comeback, for laughing at everything, and for having the courage to tell me "Honey, you ain't never gonna git a man with that floral couch!"

Trudy Menear for endless hours of typing, for listening to my ramblings, and for your constant stream of great ideas.

To my little family Johnny, Aubry, Todd, Christian, Joey, and Jack for your support and love. You know me better than anyone does; you love me more than anyone could; and you've given me more joy than I deserve.

To Al Pylinski for believing in me long before anyone else, for your generosity and love, and mostly for the truest of friendships.

Above all, I thank my Lord Jesus Christ for every breath and every step I take, for the direction You have given me, for the whispers that keep me on track, for the wisdom of Your Word, and for an amazing feeling of Peace. I can do nothing without You, but, oh my goodness, look what happens when I'm on Team Jesus! All Glory and Praise to You, Oh Lord.

Ti amo!

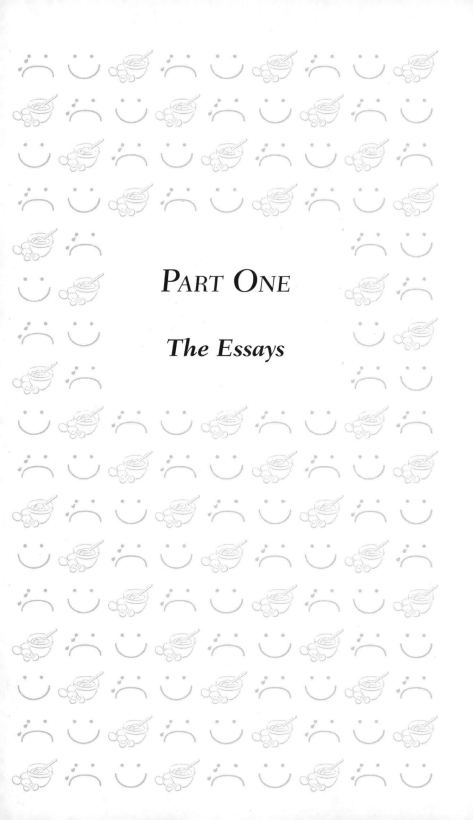

PART ONE

The Essays

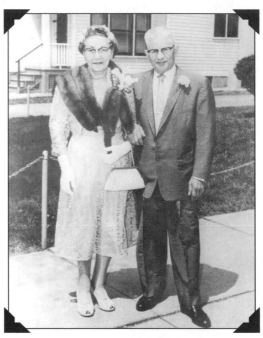

Grandma and Grandpa Conte

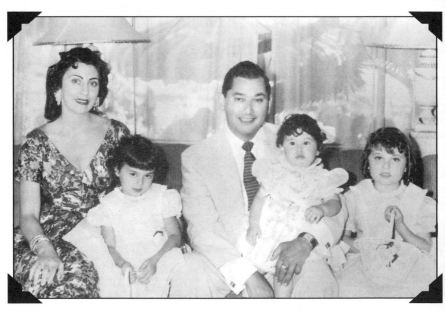

Mom, Yvonne, Daddy, Jacquelyn, and Donnarae
(Anna Marie had not yet been born)

La *Famiglia*
(The Family)

412 Ashland Avenue

Freshly picked tomatoes magically became sauce on the stove. Billows of steam escaped from pots as men smoked cigars and laughed loudly. Various sizes of children ran through the old house and women talked about the weather. One small black and white television called out the score. Someone retrieved a pan of golden crisp chicken, carrots, and potatoes from the oven and bottles of deep red homemade wine found their way to the linen covered table. Gramma Conte's kitchen was filled with luscious sounds and aromas and always with so many people. Every one of us dressed in our best clothes. This was Sunday.

Children had to sit in the kitchen at Gramma's breakfast nook. We loved it because it was like sitting at a restaurant—four or five of us on each side all squished in together, every one of us giggling, Each with our own *mopine* tied around our neck. (a part of an old tablecloth or bedsheet that Gramma had stitched along the ends so it wouldn't tear, used as a napkin). Our little faces waited

3

to be stained with tomato sauce. But we couldn't wait to finish eating and go back to the yard to play.

We could see Grampa out in the garden in his signature fedora and three-piece suit and tie. Bent over with his head buried in the greenery, he picked tender lettuce and radishes, crisp cucumbers and onions, and only the best plum tomatoes for our salad. A stick stood firmly in the ground with long strips of cord holding pie tins as hands that would hit each other, causing a ruckus and scaring the crows away.

Nothing was ever wrong at that house. Everyone was happy. There was always enough food and enough room for everyone. The uncles told jokes and everyone laughed. Most of us kids didn't know why everyone else was laughing. We laughed anyway.

Gramma always said *ca bella*, which I guess meant that we were beautiful in her eyes anyway. She was a real Gramma with an apron and glasses and a head full of gray hair and bobby pins that seemed to be there for no real reason at all. She had black shoes that laced up the front and thick stockings that went up to just above her knees. She was always either at the stove or the sink, it seemed. When one of my uncles would stick a piece of fresh bread in the sauce or steal a perfectly shaped meatball, she would hit him on the arm. He would laugh and she would say something in Italian as he left the room with his mouth full. Then a moment later she would call to one of my aunts and say, "Taste this!" as she handed over a spoonful of sauce. I could never understand that, and I remember how funny I thought it was.

Fresh garlic and parsley from the garden hung above the sink, and bowls of tomatoes and green peppers sat like photographs on the counter. I would give anything to go back to that kitchen once more and enjoy the sounds, tastes, and aromas of 412 Ashland Avenue.

First Kiss

We laughed and squealed loudly, running out of their reach as the boys chased and teased us. The spacious four-acre yard with a swing set conveniently nestled behind the three-car garage provided us with wonderful privacy as we played in the summer sun. I jumped up onto the swing set and began to walk across the bar, hand over hand, to the middle. Scott began at the opposite end and when our little faces met in the middle he kissed me! I screamed and he screamed and we jumped down off the bar and ran. We both were guilty of wiping the kiss off of our lips and making nauseous sounds. Then we all went back to the swing set to do it over again, but this time we were joined by my sister Donnarae and Scott's brother Larry. We made a game of it, lining up at one end and then the other and meeting in the middle for a kiss followed by screams, giggles, and endless running. Larry kissed Donna and Scott kissed me. It wasn't anything like I thought it would be. I had the idea that kissing a boy would somehow make me fall madly in love forever. Truthfully, I didn't feel a thing, and besides, his face was hot and sweaty and he smelled gross.

The Family

This week I worked in Wichita, Kansas. My cousin Vinny lives there with his wife Teresa and son Andrew. Because I was in town, Vinny's dad and sister, Jimmy and Stacey, drove five hours up from Texas just to see me. It didn't matter that Jimmy recently had a hip operation or that Stacey had to take time off from work to be there. They came because we're family.

We spent most of the seventy-two hours of my visit laughing and reminiscing about the old days. We have many beautiful memories of our childhood growing up in Upstate New York surrounded by a cast of characters we called The Family. Our grandfather could be found seated at his desk in the dining room with a drink in one hand and a deck of cards in the other. Dressed in a suit and tie, his shoes were shined and he never left the house without his fedora and his beautiful smile. Our grandmother was the boss of the family if truth be told. She pretty much ran the home and the family restaurant, and grandpa seemed perfectly fine with that arrangement. Her food was legendary. No matter how my poor mother tried, no one made stuffed peppers like Gramma Conte. Her home at 412 Ashland Avenue was a safe haven for all of us. It was there in the dining room that the family gathered for every birthday, anniversary, holiday, and especially for Sunday dinner. There was always enough room for everyone and the food was abundant. I never remember a cross word or a sad moment; only the sound of aunts and uncles telling stories and laughing, dishes clinking, and an army of cousins giggling around the kitchen nook.

My cousins were like sisters and brothers to me. We ran, jumped, climbed trees, and chased each other around the yard until we were hot and sweaty—all of us in our Sunday best: the boys in little suits and ties, hair neatly cut and slicked to perfection, and the girls in party dresses, lace trimmed socks, patent leather shoes, and sausage curls with ribbons. We caught lightning bugs in jars and marveled at how they flickered. We ate fresh purple grapes right off the vine, played tickle-fish and laughed until we couldn't breath. The bigger kids looked after the little kids and someone always fell and cried as their mom cleaned up the scrape and put on a Band-Aid. We never gave a thought to what a wonderful time we were fortunate to be living in.

I knew these people would always be there for me.

I could count on them. I knew they loved me, if for no other reason but that we were and always would be family. I want my grandchildren to know that kind of security and love. I want to ensure that they have these kinds of memories. I want to know that one day long into the future, one of their cousins will travel five hours by car just to see them for a few hours because they're family.

True Friends and Italian Cheese

Out of the blue the phone call came. "It's Peggy! I'm coming to Syracuse!" The familiar sound of a dear friend was just as full of cheer as the thirteen-year-old I had met forty-six years before. Peggy O'Neil and I first met in 1965 at Saint Cyril's Academy for Girls in Danville, Pennsylvania, where she quickly became my best friend. Both of us were sent to the boarding school by our parents in the hopes of a better education and, in my case, a place where I might learn some discipline. We didn't get either, but we did create a bond that has remained strong through four husbands, five kids, and four grandchildren!

We hit all the hot spots in town today and reminisced about the past. We started our day at the farmers' market, picking out fresh tomatoes, cherries, grapes, salt potatoes, plums, and lemons from local growers. We sat in the sun and drank coffees and enjoyed a bite to eat at a small café. At the Italian import store we bought fresh mozzarella and a special imported vinegar to go with our ripe red tomatoes. On the way home we stopped at Columbus Bakery for fresh bread—the same bakery my father took me to every Sunday after church. We would buy three loaves of bread: two for our dinner and one to eat out of the bag on the way home. So in honor of my dad, Peggy and I bought one for dinner and pulled the fresh, soft, still warm bread from the second bag and ate it with much delight. Next stop: the Italian deli next door for some unbelievably delicious smoked provolone! Yum! Just smelling the aroma of these priceless Italian specialties brings me back to my childhood when things seemed simpler, life was to be enjoyed, and Peggy and I giggled in the last row of room 416 in Sr. Mary Paul's Latin class.

Peggy and I have had a wonderful visit, reminiscing and visiting with friends and family. We've laughed a lot. There's something absolutely comforting about connecting with long-time friends. They know you. They know your heart. It's almost as if they are a part of your soul, the very fabric of who you are. Make it a point to visit with old friends. Take that trip, make the call, and reconnect. Just do it. You'll be so glad you did.

In 1965 we were two mischievous little thrill seekers and we drove our poor parents crazy. Today Peggy is the mayor of Deerfield Beach, Florida, and I'm a keynote speaker and author. (Side note to parents of unruly children: It all works out in the end!)

Grateful Lessons Learned

I wouldn't call myself a disobedient child, but in our family there were three little darling young ladies and one spirited, often devilish little girl. No matter how naughty I was, Daddy never hit me. He couldn't. His swollen arthritic hands carried too much pain; it really would have "hurt him, more than it did me." Instead, he taught me that when you do good things, good things happen to you.

"Turn that TV off and get these beds made up." He only said it once. I could hear his footsteps above my head as my hero Popeye saved his sweetheart Olive from the horrible Brutus once again. "Yuk yuk yuk yuk yuk..." I loved the way that skinny character laughed. My giggles were soon the only sounds I could hear and my bed lay crumpled and unmade.

Daddy decided to take us girls to Shoppingtown in Dewitt later that afternoon. He handed each of my sisters a crisp new $20 bill, just for being good. My sisters didn't seem to notice the door of the car as it closed with me still inside. He simply said, "Vonnie, I need you to stay with me today." I sat alone in that big back seat and watched my sisters' smiling faces disappear into Dey Brothers Department Store as we pulled away from the curb. I felt so left out.

Later that night Daddy called my older sister Donnarae to his knee. With a little squeeze and a wet kiss on her cheek, he proudly said, "I've got the most beautiful four daughters in the whole world." The daughter adored walked away a princess while I wore the face of deep sorrow. I knew I had disappointed him that morning. Just knowing that was my punishment.

The very next day, I couldn't wait to get out of bed so I could smooth the covers and fluff the pillows. With every wrinkle smoothed and every corner tucked, I waited in anticipation for a glimpse of his face as he passed my room. All he did was wink. *Yes!* I'm back in his good graces! On top of the ferris wheel of daughterdom. Daddy winked at me. He was proud of me, and that was everything to me.

He was a good man and a great dad. Nearly sixty years later, I'm grateful for the lessons he taught me. I'm grateful for the woman I have become because of him. And of course, I always make my bed as soon as my feet hit the carpet.

Scent of a Father

Shopping cart wheels rolled on the pavement and parents and children filled their trunks with bags of soda, meats and vegetables. It was an ordinary morning until that scent permeated the air and for one instant I thought he was near. My head lifted. I filled my lungs with air and my eyes searched the parking lot. There it was—that scent for one split second—and then it was gone. The sweet smell of a man's cigar had taken me back twelve years to a time before my father's generous heart stopped beating; before his glorious smile was taken. I sat back in my car and tears began to well. I took a deep breath and remembered how he loved us all individually and collectively, how he made us all feel special and unique, how he held his family together through good times and difficult ones. I missed him. I took a deep breath and walked into the store grateful for the smell of a man's cigar and the gift it gave me in that moment.

Stand Up Straight

Recently, I had to go to the Department of Motor Vehicles to return my license plates. People were waiting, filling the room—some sitting, some standing. This motley group of drivers sat hunched over reading papers, legs propped up on backpacks, and arms stretched across the backs of chairs. One young girl had her head propped up in the palm of her hand as if it were just too heavy to stay up on its own. I looked at the people who were standing in line alongside of me. Lifting weight from the left foot to the right, men shifted anxiously forward. Ladies moved their heavy purses from shoulder to shoulder, causing them to lean slightly from one side to the other. Some people propped one foot on the bar under the counter when they finally got there, as if that was some sort of reward for standing in line so long. I saw many different sizes of people in all sorts of positions, yet rarely did I see anyone standing with perfect posture like I do. Like a ballerina waiting for my turn to dance,

I stand tall and straight with an attitude of certainty. My mother taught me to stand that way, and I'm so grateful for it.

All those evenings in the living room, walking around in a circle with a book balanced on top of my head, have given me not just good posture, but an air of confidence and poise that others don't seem to have.

My mom, my sisters, and I laughed together and we tried to out-do one another. It was a game to see who could walk the furthest and balance the book the longest. It was all just fun back then for us girls. However, Mom knew exactly what she was doing. She was teaching us girls lifelong lessons. I'm delighted that I stand tall no matter where I am. I thank my mother for coaching me to be confident and secure and to walk into a room as if I own it!

Wrestling Match and Exercise

Ten legs of different sizes and shapes seemed to be growing out of the living room floor. Each pair of limbs worked intensely—doing the "bicycle" as fast as they could. There was my mother at the head of the class showing us girls how to have shapely, strong legs like hers. Somehow she always managed to stay up longer than the rest of us, peddling fast and with precise form. I wanted to be like my mother so I tried very hard to keep up with her. I think that's how the wresting matches between her and me started out. She always seemed to get me pinned down. No matter how hard I tried to pin her, I just never made it.

Those were pleasurable times on the living room floor. I think about it sometimes and wish I could go back just one more time and laugh like that again on the floor with my mother and sisters. Annie always ended up crying at some point. She was just too little to realize that mom and I were just having fun. Mom really wore me out. I thank her for spending time with me, for laughing with me, and for giving me some of the most wonderful memories.

Curls

Sitting still for very long was always dreadfully difficult for me. That made it especially hard for my mom to force my pin-straight hair to coil around her finger. A black hairpin would hold it in place for the night, setting her fingers free to work on the next rebellious thread of hair. She spent hours coaxing strands of my fine lifeless locks to become delightful dancing ringlets. I can still smell the sweet clean aroma of the Nestlé's hair tonic she used to force the curls into place, hoping to give them bounce and shine. My sisters' hair always came out better than mine. I suppose the fact that sitting still seemed easier for them had something to do with it.

One day, after having had enough of this nightly ritual, I stood in front of the full-length mirror in my room and one by one I chopped the long curls off. It was not an act of defiance but rather one of comfort. I just wanted a hairstyle more in line with my personality. I wore a "pixie" haircut for the remainder of my childhood, which made me stand out from my sisters. From then on I felt like the ugly duckling next to my three very pretty and always lovely coiffed siblings. I still haven't learned to sit still. What I *have* learned is that my mother just wanted me to be pretty. She wanted to do whatever it took to help me to become a fine young lady. And as hard as I may have made it for her to accomplish her goal, she succeeded. Thank you, Mom, for helping me to become a fine young lady…even one with a pixie haircut.

Popcorn and Ed Sullivan

Sunday night meant popcorn, Ed Sullivan, and his "really big shew." With a bowl of Mom's pan-popped, still warm popcorn in front of me, perfectly salted with just the right amount of real butter, I watched and listened. No popcorn has ever smelled as delicious or tasted as good. The best part of it all was that I could count on enjoying this ritual every Sunday night without fail.

The first time I heard the Italian puppet mouse Topo Gigio say, "Eddie, keesa me goo' night," the first time I laughed at José Jiménez, and the very first time I got a glimpse of my beloved John, Paul, George, and Ringo, my family was enjoying it all with me. While we munched on Mom's perfectly popped corn, Elvis swiveled that famous pelvis and June Taylor and her Toastettes kicked their high-healed legs in the air. We laughed together on Sunday nights around the television set—it was part of our family tradition.

Up in our beds after the lights went out, I would turn to my sister Donna and in the voice of Señor Wences's talking box, I would say, "S'a' right?" and she would answer, "S'a' right!" Our little girl giggles lasted long into the night.

I can't seem to watch much television anymore without a bowl of popcorn in front of me. I never make it as enjoyable as my mother did, but with every bite I think of how she made our house a home. I think of the time she took to do special things, like pop us our corn and laugh with us on Sunday nights in front of the TV.

Flowers, Flowers, and More Flowers

Smiling yellow daffodils and jonquils, dazzling red tulips and vivid purple and blue heather fill my flower bed in the spring of the year. They begin to peek through the earth and surround my house with color, and I think of my mother. I watched her tend to her garden and shine with pride when she brought her luscious roses into the house. I noticed that she couldn't wait to get out there in the spring of the year and get the ground ready. Somehow every year she turned a chaotic brown bed of weeds into a heavenly scented paradise. My mother gave me the gift of love for flowers. She taught me how to plant the bulbs and told me the mystery about the eggshells and coffee grounds. With each flower that grins at me in the morning, I think of her—even when I'm pulling the weeds away so my flowers can grow. My mother's love of the garden has made my world a little bit more beautiful.

Blue-Eyed Princess

There was something I always thought about when I was growing up. In the bathroom at 30 Draycott Street, I spent hours looking in the mirror at my face and wishing I looked more like my mother. Everyone always told me I looked like Dad's side of the family, but I wanted to look like the blue-eyed princess that was my mother. She was the most beautiful woman I had ever seen.

On any given day of my childhood, she looked like a movie star or a princess. No one else's mom could even compare to her. Thick, glossy, dark auburn hair brushed against her creamy white skin and it took my breath away. Her eyes sparkled like blue diamonds and they still do today. I have always been very proud of my mother. When I was growing up, I knew that of all my friends, I had the most beautiful mother.

Now I find myself looking at pictures of her, trying desperately to see a resemblance. Recently one of my friends saw a picture of my mother, my daughter Aubry, and me, and she said, "Oh my, you all look alike." It was the sweetest thing she could have said. I keep that picture on my dresser now. I'm very happy that, finally, after all these years, someone thinks I look like my beautiful mom.

The Order of a Meal

The typical meal at our house on a Sunday consisted of several courses. The *aperitivo* was a drink we offered people the minute they came in the door (a little chilled vermouth with a twist of lemon peel sort of got you in the mood for the feast that was about to come).

Once we all sat down at the table and said Grace, a glass of red wine was raised; the toast was given, *"Salute!"* and out came the *antipasto,* which was always a huge oval platter of attractive Italian meats and cheeses, olives, anchovies, ceci beans, cherry peppers, and other delights, all laying perfectly on a bed of fresh crisp romaine lettuce. Oftentimes we would then have a nice bowl of homemade soup, something light with lots of broth, and always a pasta of some sort with a red sauce. The sauce was made with sausage, pork, or veal, and sometimes chicken.

After these dishes were taken off the table, we would enjoy the *primo piatto,* or the main course. Mom would make a roast or chicken with potatoes and vegetables. Then came many different cheeses, nuts, and fruits, along with strong coffee and *dolce,* our dessert. This usually took us about two and half hours to complete. We ate slowly. We talked and laughed. We took our time and really enjoyed it.

We were used to this. We expected it. However, the first time I brought my prospective husband home to meet the family, we quickly learned that we were from very different cultures. When my father poured the vermouth and offered it to him, he asked my dad for a beer. I cringed, but my father, being the gentleman he was, ordered me to go down to the refrigerator in the cellar and get him a beer. Once we sat at the table he picked over the antipasto as if he were confused. I was beginning to feel sorry for him. When he saw the pasta, his eyes lit up, and he said with a big grin, "Now, *that's* something I recognize!" I remember that my mother and father glanced at each other, and I wondered what in the world they were thinking.

Here's where this story takes a very bad turn: Each of us took a small portion of pasta to taste and passed the dish along. When it got to my husband-to-be, he filled his dinner plate with pasta. I mean, it was piled high! And then he committed a mortal sin: He cut his pasta with a knife into small bite-size bits! I thought my mother would faint. The rest of us twirled our pasta onto our forks and watched him cut the pasta as if he were cutting up a piece of steak. He never noticed our dismay.

We were all done and ready for the main course, but we had to wait until he was finished with his mound of cut-up pasta. It took him an agonizing twenty minutes. My father began to get impatient and drum his fingers on the tablecloth as he waited.

Finally, we took the dishes off the table and mom brought a platter filled with roasted lamb and another brimming with vegetables and potatoes, and we all began to eat—all except our poor guest of honor. He was just totally confused. He finally told us that he thought the pasta *was* the meal and couldn't figure out why we ate so little. He had never heard of eating so many different things at one meal. We all had a great laugh over that and to this day we still talk about it. My father and my (since divorced) husband, actually became good friends. I know they grew to respect each other. This was a great lesson for me. People are different. We all come from many different backgrounds. It is always glorious when

I see two people who have almost nothing in common become friends and treat each other with respect. These two men always did.

Life Well Lived

Long before women burned their bras and raised their voices for equal rights, one woman quietly paved the way. The choices she made in her life taught her four daughters, seven granddaughters, and four great-granddaughters that a women can do anything she wants to do with her life. All you have to do is really, really want it and it's yours.

It was 1934. Nine-year-old Angela, the seventh child in a family of eleven children, was at her dance class at the local YMCA. Her dance teacher asked if any of the girls in the class could sing. Five girls quickly raised their hands and the teacher asked to hear each one. Angela couldn't wait for her turn. The teacher heard her crystal-clear voice and invited her to sing for the Rotary Club. Angela said she would love to, but would have to ask her mother's permission. That night she wore her beautiful confirmation dress and sang for the Rotary Club in town. She said, "Singing made me feel special and I loved it!" Angela had found her calling.

After her "debut" at the Rotary Club, she began getting invitations to sing for various functions around town. She was the only child in the adult choir at church and sang all the solos in Latin. She entered a talent contest at the Midnight Movie House and won first prize, which led her to sing live on the radio in Hazleton, a nearby town. Before she turned ten, it seemed this little girl knew exactly what she wanted to do with her life. In an era when little girls were taught to cook and clean and were expected to get married and have a man take care of them, Angela had other ideas.

Soon after graduation, she and her sisters, Marie and Ginny, left home and shared an apartment in Baltimore. While her sisters went to work for Eastern Aircraft, Angela secured two agents and sang in night clubs and hotels around town. She was booked quickly and her singing profession was in full swing. She enjoyed an exciting career as "Vonnie Blue," and was the featured singer in venues up and down the East Coast. She especially enjoyed working with the big bands in Atlantic City and on the Boardwalk. Vonnie Blue (Angela) was a hit!

Just when her career seemed to be at its peek, she met Frank Conte, a handsome, charismatic, and persistent man. It was 1946 and she was the featured act at the Kirk Grill on Blandina Street in Utica. They fell in love and were married in 1947. Angela soon gave up her thriving career on the stage and assisted her husband with his growing business. He was vice president in charge of sales at Permanent Stainless Steel Corporation and employed sixty cookware salesmen. Angela became president and creator of the Permanent Stainless Steel Women's Club for the wives of these men. She held regular meetings and created a monthly magazine telling about the activities of those in the club. This was a very progressive thing for a woman to be doing in the early '50s. She did all this while raising four daughters and caring for her husband, who was stricken with rheumatoid arthritis soon after they were married.

In 1960, the family moved from Utica to Syracuse. Angela never lost her love of music and began to sing at Holy Cross Church in Dewitt as the soloist for weddings and funerals and all the Latin masses.

Angela was and still is a great example to all women. We have the opportunity to make choices in our lives. Angela never made excuses, she never said it's too hard, she never complained, she never blamed. She took responsibility for her life. She knew what she wanted and she went for it. I am proud to call her Mom.

Frank W. Conte,
World War II Navy Veteran

At the New York State Fair in Syracuse, there's a Veterans War Memorial Walk. My father has a brick in that walk. I couldn't wait to find the memorial and search for my father's name among the many sailors in the Navy section. After what seemed like an eternity, I saw "...W. Conte" barely peeking out from under a man's shoe. Standing on top of the "Frank" was a very large man. Patiently, I waited for him to move. He just stood there with his back to me, not knowing he was standing on my father's brick. I don't know why, but tears began to well up in my eyes right there on a Sunday afternoon in the midst of thousands of strangers at the New York State Fair. I tapped the man's shoulder and in a frail voice I said, "Excuse me, sir...you're standing on my father's brick." Immediately he moved away and I dropped down to touch the brick. I gently moved my fingers over his name. "Frank W. Conte, United States Navy, WW II Electrician." That was all I needed. I walked across the busy sidewalk to an area under three flagpoles. Alone on a bench under a beautiful tree, I watched the flags wave proudly in the wind as if to salute the soldiers, and I thought about my father.

There was a veterans' band playing loud, happy music, and someone was singing. People were everywhere, but somehow I felt like it was just me and my daddy on that bench. I looked across the way to where the memorial was. Knowing how proud he was to serve his country, it was such a comfort to know my father's name would be there forever. Thousands of people will come here every year and walk past his name.

Then I thought, How could it be that he has been gone for over fifteen years and I feel like he is still with me? So often I think of him. When I am working, I'm remembering all that he taught me about business and success. When I am with my children, I'm thinking how wonderful a parent he was and how easily he taught me to love. I think of how comfortable he was in the kitchen and I can hear him telling me, "The secret to good clam sauce is the anchovies!"

What will my children think of when they think of me? What kind of example am I? What have I taught them? We have each been given a certain amount of time. We can do with it whatever we want. But when we are gone, whatever we have done with that time will live on in the minds of the people whose lives we have touched. My father taught me many life lessons, but the one that has made the most difference in my life is what he taught me after he passed away. I want to leave my children with good memories. I want to give them something to be proud of. Long after I am gone, I want them to be able to sit on a park bench and realize that life counts for something, that what we do with the time we are given matters. I want my children to know that the most important part of a person's life is how they touched the lives of others.

Answered Questions

While she slept, I watched her breath. Her small body moving a bit with each intake of air, and I questioned everything. Will I be able to take care of her if she gets sick? Will I make the right choices? Will I be too strict? Not strict enough?

I waited quietly while she danced the ballet and wondered, Was I patient? Did she eat enough today? Am I a good example? With every birthday and Christmas, was I spoiling her? Would she learn to be appreciative and generous or expect to have everything given to her? What was I teaching her about relationships, trust, love? Should I let her watch that show, go to that movie, have that experience? No one ever teaches you how to be a parent. You never really know if you are doing it right. You just love your kids and pray real hard.

With the stunning beauty and grace of a princess, she picked up her simple bouquet of white daisies and opened the door. A strong, confidant, generous, kind woman walked toward me, reached out and hugged my neck. "This is the happiest day of my life," she whispered, "Thank you Momma."

And the wondering was over.

Thirty Years of Love

Thirty years ago I took my children, Aubry and Johnny, to a free show at a mall to see Gordon, a character they had come to know from the children's show, *Sesame Street*. Johnny had a great time singing and dancing with all the other children, but it was my daughter Aubry's reaction to Gordon that took my breath away. She was mesmerized by him. She didn't dance and sing like the other children. Instead she just stood there staring at Gordon, watching him intently, as if she were trying to figure something out. I had never seen her so taken by anyone before. After the show, all the other children were being silly, pushing and shoving each other, laughing and all worked up from the excitement of the show and the sugar. Aubry stood like a ballerina, just watching her hero sign his name on his glossy eight-by-tens. It was interesting to watch how she methodically maneuvered her way up to the front of the line to get his autograph and have her picture taken with him. My daughter absolutely loved Gordon.

Last week, when I read in the paper that Gordon would be at the Palace Theater here in Syracuse, I thought it would be wonderful to take my grandson Joey to see him. I wanted to see how he would react to his mother's childhood idol.

We arrived at the Palace an hour early and, lo and behold, Gordon was just getting out of the WCNY van in front of the theater. Joey and I approached him and asked if we could take a picture. He was as caring and gentle as he had been the first time I met him so many years ago. I showed him the picture of him with Aubry that I had taken, and he actually said, "Where was that taken?" I said, "In Chattanooga, about 1979." He smiled and said, "I remember that visit to Chattanooga." Then he gazed at the picture of Aubry and then took a good look at Joey. He patted Joey on the top of his head and said with his signature grin, "And this is her little boy? How about that!"

I found Roscoe Orman to be every bit as kind as the character that has become a fixture on *Sesame Street*. Meeting him again on that sidewalk was all I really needed to make it worth my time and the price of the ticket.

Joey was excited when we entered the theater and saw the big picture of all the *Sesame Street* characters on the screen and heard the music blaring. We settled in on the very front row and waited patiently. I was remembering how much this had meant to Aubry, and was secretly hoping Joey would have the same reaction. When the show started, Joey jumped right in and danced and sang and clapped his hands. He had a ball, front and center, right in front of Gordon. Joey was all boy. He was just there to have fun. I was a bit disappointed that he wasn't enthralled with Gordon like his mom was. I sat in my seat and got all teary-eyed just thinking of my daughter and how she loved this man. When Gordon sang a sweet song about wanting a child, called "If I Had a Kid Like You," I had to get the Kleenex out. This man had been a big part of my daughter's childhood. He helped her learn to count, taught her the ABCs, and showed her how to dance and sing. He had been a strong male role model and I felt like this was a very full-circle moment for me.

Once the show was over and Joey was strapped in his car seat, we chatted a bit about the day. I asked him what was the best part of the day and his response was the potato chips he got to pick out for himself at lunch. It wasn't the response I had hoped for.

After a few minutes of silence, Joey spoke. "I'd like to go see Gordon again tomorrow, Nonni." I replied, "Oh, honey, Gordon has to go back to *Sesame Street*. That was the only time we can see him except on TV." Little Joey thought a minute and then took a big sigh and said with a smile, "Oh, well, that's okay. I can always go there in my dreams!" I cried all the way home. He is his mama's kid.

Aubry Lynne Ludington

A good daughter is like a good piece of writing: truthful, poetic, polished, poignant, full of life. I have seen you walk across the stage, intent on your errand, and it was like watching a sound become visible, as if not your voice, but your motion, said, "I will do this for my life." To be your mother is to be grateful for the rest of my life for having had the privilege. Who you have become is grander than anything I prayed for, much more than my greatest hope, and far superior than I could have ever imagined.

Johnny Frances Ludington

I laughed today when a friend was talking about her little boy and his interest in bugs. When my son Johnny was about four, he had a milk jug filled with caterpillars. I made him keep them outside. It rained really hard one night and Johnny cried because he wanted to bring his bugs inside. I explained that they were used to being outside and refused to let them come in. Little Johnny waited until I went to bed. Then he went out to the porch and brought his bugs in. He set the jug on his pillow and went to sleep. The bugs all crawled out and as Johnny slept he squished them all by accident. He woke up to a messy bunch of dead bugs. He cried for days. He had a pet roly-poly bug that he named Fred. I woke up one morning and saw Fred on the kitchen floor. I didn't have my glasses on and thought it was a roach (we lived in the South at the time). As I ran to pounce on the "roach," Johnny cried, "No! That's Fred!" It was too late. Fred was already murdered and again Johnny cried for days. As John grew older he would do things like catch a fly inside the house and let it go outside to save its life. I thought he was so weird. Johnny is thirty-six years old now and lives in California. He is just about the kindest young man I know. He still cries whenever an animal is hurt and he has a heart of gold. I wouldn't change him for anything.

Peace

We always want what we don't have until we get it,
then we want what we had.

The house is still except for the ticking of the clock and the hum of the furnace. The chairs sit empty at the dining room table and the lace cloth waits neatly in the drawer. I would love some company, but it seems my family has outgrown the need to enjoy Sunday dinner together. My sister Donna and her family are going to start their holiday shopping, my daughter and her family plan to go to a movie, and my sister Jacky and her crew decided to clean out the cellar. I wish I had the busy lives everyone else seems to have. No one has time for Sunday dinner because they have filled the day with other important things to do. Having my house full of kids, noise, and commotion somehow represents home to me. The joy of someone snatching a freshly fried chicken cutlet from the pan or dipping a hunk of fresh bread into my sauce is just a fading memory. There is nothing to clean because no one ever messes anything up! This place is so quiet, I expect Jesus to walk in and tell me heaven called and they want their peace back. Feeling rather sorry for myself, I decide to make a big pot of sauce and some meatballs simply to have the familiar aroma greet me when I come in from church. While I'm there, I pray for God to help me to appreciate what I have.

Upon my return from church, the blinking light on the phone is a welcome sign. My daughter changed plans and will come for dinner. They are bringing the dog, too. Terrific! Oh, this is wonderful! The lace tablecloth comes out of the drawer and the china, silver, and crystal take their place at the dining room table, and everything seems right with the world. I begin to cook up some pork chops and potatoes and the phone rings again. This time it's Jacky who reconsiders. Five more places are set at the table. I head to the bakery for some freshly baked bread. Soon the house is filled with family. Children run through the rooms, the ball game blares from the TV, cheese is being grated, and sauce is being poured. Just as we sit down to eat, Donna and her family surprise us at the door. We move the kids into the kitchen to make room for the grown-ups at the dining room table. I'm so happy! It smells like home. It sounds like home. Ah... the noise, the commotion, and the disorder—how blissfully wonderful! We spend hours around the table talking, laughing, and eating. Little Joseph gets more on the floor than in his mouth. I'll get it with the vacuum later. This is just what I had hoped for. That sauce stain will probably come out if I soak it. I'm exhausted, but this is what I wanted, right? Oh, my goodness, don't these kids ever stop yelling and running? I'm exhausted. Too tired to say anything, I just watch as the dog buries something in the garden. I can't hear myself think. Why do they all have to talk at once? I box up the leftovers and send them out the door with love. Children are buckled in. Kisses. Hugs. Car doors slam shut. Down the drive they go. It was so nice to have the family over.

Every cup is back in the cabinet and every chair is in its place. Ahhhhhhhh! Order, quiet, peace. The ticking of the clock. The hum of the furnace. I sit with a cup of tea and enjoy the silence. You just don't realize how great it is until it's gone.

Go Play!

It's Memorial Day and I spent the better part of the day relaxing on my sun porch, reading and writing and enjoying the peacefulness of my home. My table was set, fresh cupcakes sat proudly on the cake stand, the fruit was cut, and water was boiling for the salt potatoes. But the atmosphere changed with a knock at the door. My two young grandsons, Joseph, three, and Jack, one, came for a picnic accompanied by my son-in-law Todd. My daughter was away at a meeting. They were here just two and half hours. Yet I am completely and utterly exhausted. I must have gone in and out of the back door at the very least thirty-seven times—bringing some fruit out to them, running in to get some napkins, out again to get the ball out of the garden and in again to check the potatoes. I heard my name called over forty times: "Nonni, come play! Nonni, I need help! Nonni, I can't reach! Nonni, I want bubbles! Nonni! Nonni!"

We dragged all the toys out of the shed: the kiddy lawn mower, the rocking horse, hula-hoops, balls, rackets, toy shopping carts, and, in a last attempt to amuse them, the bouncy ball house, accompanied by two hundred plastic balls. At last, dinner was ready and we came in to eat. Along with potatoes, cheeseburgers, and salad, there was crying, spilled juice, and a lot of up and down, getting this or that, and a major negotiation to eat just one more bite. While Todd and I finished our dinner, Jack and Joe managed to get every toy out of the toy box in the living room and spread it all across the living room floor.

After dinner we went outside and blew bubbles for ten minutes before they gathered up their stuff and headed home.

I don't remember these kinds of visits when I was a kid. I remember that the grown-ups sat leisurely around the dining room table sipping coffee and having civil conversations, while we kids enjoyed running around the back yard playing tag. We got an old can and kicked it around the yard; we climbed the tree; or we simply sat on the grass and made flower chains. There were no big plastic toys or ball houses and no one came running out of the house when one of us fell down. We simply got up and kept on running. We never needed Mom or Dad or Nonni to come out and play with us. We knew how to play and we did it all day long. When dinner time came we ate what was put in front of us—we never asked what it was; we just ate it. We never even thought of playing in the living room—that was where the grown-ups sat. After dinner, we went back outside and played until dark, when sometimes we'd catch lightning bugs in jars.

How did life change so drastically? When did parents begin to monitor every single thing a child does? We buy them the latest newfangled toy or gadget in an attempt to give them something to do. In the process, they have become a society of children who don't know how to amuse themselves, who don't know how to just play outside in the yard.

I love my little grandsons, and the next time they come over I am going to do my darnedest to run and jump and chase and tumble and fall and get up again and run some more. I want to teach them the fine art of simply going out in the yard to play.

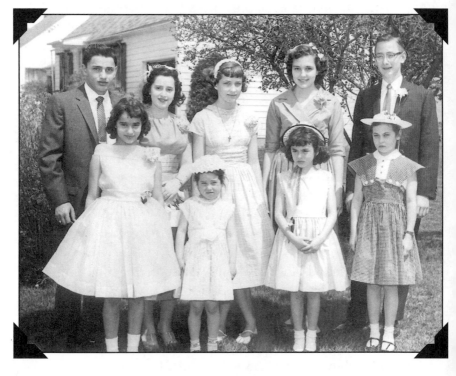

Cousins
Jimmy, Marilyn, Joyce, Carla, Tony,
Nancy, Jacky, Yvonne, Donnarae
(Carolyn and Anna Marie had not yet been born)

Travel

Travelers Will Eat Anything

Today I ate a cheeseburger. I never eat cheeseburgers, but I was hungry and the choices were slim. The cheeseburger was microwaved a bit too long, making the bun the consistency of damp cardboard and the burger itself was more like rubber than an actually piece of meat. I ate it anyway. I can't think of any situation in my life where I would eat such a thing, but I was on a train and I had just paid ten dollars for it. I bought what I thought was a better choice of chips because they were called "Terra Exotic Vegetable Chips" and the bag looked healthy. Halfway through the bag, I thought, Gee, this is sort of like eating glass. The chips were so hard and brittle and they cracked loudly when I bit into them. Even though they were tasteless, I ate the entire bag.

I eat snacks on a plane that I would never consider eating at home, like a bag of four tiny pretzels. Why would you eat four tiny pretzels? It just makes you thirsty, and we've all read about how filthy the ice is on planes. Then we are forced to drink a soda with no ice. So you are eating four tiny pretzels and a warm Diet Pepsi. Why? I don't have the answer. It's not satisfying in any way, except I feel like I have to take what they give me on a plane because they screwed me on the damned luggage charge. I want to feel like I'm getting something free.

Last night I was in a hotel that had a microwave in the lobby. I stopped at a gas station and saw a bowl of microwave macaroni and cheese. You guessed it! I bought it and took it to the lobby and nuked it. Back in the privacy of my room I mixed the powdered, pretend cheese with the macaroni and I ate it. It was horrible. Every last speck of it.

Why do we eat things when we're traveling that would never enter our mouths if we were anywhere else? I think it's because we're trapped. We feel that if we don't eat what's put in front of us, we may never get another meal. I'm not sure, but I think it must be my mother's fault. When I was growing up, she said, "You eat what's on your plate. People are starving in China." At the time, I didn't know where China was, and I didn't know why they were starving there, but I did what my mother told me and I ate what was put in front of me. Some habits never die.

Just Plane Funny

I once had the inside of a window on a plane fall into my lap just before lift off. I panicked and called for an attendant. We were already taxiing down the runway and the attendants were prepared for takeoff. After several attempts to get their attention, I just held the window straight up over my head and yelled, "Hey, don't go yet!" Still, no one up front heard me. I quickly unbuckled my seat belt and ran up the aisle with the window in my hand, yelling, "Don't go yet! My window fell out!" Some passengers were laughing and others were gasping. Long story short—they stopped the plane and two repairmen came aboard to fix the window. They said it was just "cosmetic," and that we could have flown safely without fixing it. I thought, "Hey, if the window falls out, what's next? The wings fall off?

The interesting part of this story is that several flights earlier, a man sitting next to me had a prosthetic leg that was coming off. He was struggling with it, trying to get it back in place. I offered to help him. I got on my knees in front of him and carefully adjusted the leg to get it back on and comfortable for him. He thanked me and asked me if I was a nurse. I said, "No, I'm a comedian." The rest of the passengers on the plane cracked up.

The flight attendant on the plane with the broken window recognized me and jokingly said, "I know you— you're the gal that tried to rip that guys leg off on one of my other flights!" He then turned to the passengers behind me and said, "Watch her, she's trouble!" I guess what I learned from each episode is that no matter what's happening, if you add a little humor to the mix, it just makes it easier to get through.

West New York

I presented the keynote address at West New York High School in New Jersey, situated along the bank of the Hudson River facing New York City near the George Washington Bridge. There are 55,000 people who live in West New York, which is only one square mile. Yep—55,000 people in one square mile. Hard to imagine. Everyone— and I mean everyone—I came in contact with was an absolute delight. You would think people who live in such a crowded environment would be grumpy, pushy people, but that was not the case at all. You would expect that when the cookie break started, people would push and shove to get to the table first and that it would be a fight to get a seat. Instead, they patiently waited in line and happily chatted with one another to pass the time. They were loving, genuine people who all live and work in this one square mile. They said it was like a small town where everyone knows you—shop keepers call you by name. My experience there was such a pleasure.

The ride home, however, was a horse of a different color. The plane was full—not a seat to be had. We had an entire high school ball team, one crying baby, a dog who would not stop barking, and a cat who threw up several times. It was lovely. The part of the trip that sent most passengers over the top was that we sat on the tarmac for two hours before takeoff. Nice. I found it so interesting how people reacted to what was happening. I sat next to what seemed like a completely normal lady and her daughter returning from a vacation in Florida. Thirty minutes into the wait, she snapped. She actually stood up and yelled, "Can we at least get some snacks back here if you're gonna make us wait like this?" I couldn't believe it. She continued shouting at the poor flight attendant, "Hey! How 'bout some snacks? Pass out the snacks!" I offered her a piece of sugar-free gum. That's all I had. The boys on the ball team played cards, tossed a ball around, and shared their copy of *Hustler*, while each one of them talked as if they were the only ones on the plane. The baby continued to cry and the dog to bark, however the cat stopped throwing up during the second hour. I really enjoyed observing the passengers around me. It's great research for future presentations on human behavior. I bet money that ninety percent of these people, if they were at home, would be planted firmly in front of their television sets anyway, so I really found it interesting that when they were forced to watch the television on the back of each seat, it pissed them off.

The bottom line is that we all arrived at our destination safe and sound and that went on my joy list once I got home. We are such a spoiled society. Any inconvenience and we whine like little children. We had an opportunity to enjoy a movie, catch up on our prayers, read a good book, or get to know the person next to us. Most, however, chose to complain. It was a very good lesson for me. From now on I want to pay attention to my own reaction to inconvenience. When I am short-tempered, impatient, and unkind to people who may not go as fast as I want them to, I will think of the joyful people I met on that one square mile in West New York. I'll take a deep breathe and relax.

Leaving Las Vegas—No Easy Task

My flight was to leave Vegas at 11:15 A.M. The airport shuttle driver was late picking me up at Planet Hollywood and then took his sweet time stopping at three other hotels before dropping me at the airport at 10:45. I raced to get my boarding pass and then hurried through security. I managed to get the gate attendant to move my seat from 24D to 12A. At least I'd be getting off the plane a few minutes earlier in Cleveland. With only a twenty-minute wait between connections, I didn't want to miss my flight to Syracuse. It had been a long work week and I was eager to come home.

All my rushing around proved to be a waste of energy. At 3:10 P.M. I was still at the Vegas airport waiting patiently as my flight was delayed, and delayed, and delayed. My new flight was scheduled to leave Vegas at 11:30 P.M., connecting in Cleveland and getting me home at 10:15 the next morning. Such is the glamorous life of the motivational keynote speaker. I guess this is why we get the big bucks. This is the part of my job no one thinks about when they are trying to get me to reduce my speaker fee by half. I tell you: patience—it really takes patience.

One of the benefits of being forced to sit still for twelve hours is that it offers the opportunity to enjoy one of my favorite pastimes—people watching. Two young women stood at the gate counter. One Asian with short black hair and a bad complexion, who I'll call Agent #1, and an average-looking black women wearing an "I love Jesus" ID holder, who I'll call Agent #2. Each woman was doing the same job, searching for flights for the 180 people who were told the plane had been struck by lightning on the way in and that our flight to Cleveland would be delayed, causing most of us to miss our connecting flights.

As the crowd grew angry, the gals went to work finding connecting flights from Cleveland to our final destinations. Granted, this was not an easy task, but I noticed something interesting about the Gate Agents and the results of their very different demeanors. Agent #1 huffed and puffed her way through the task, raising her voice to passengers and repeating the same irritating mantra, "I'm doing the best I can ma'am!" and never looking anyone in the eye. She frequently got on the speaker to say, "Please do not crowd around the counter. We will call you by name when we are ready to redirect your flight. Do not come to the counter unless your name has been called." Each time she slammed the receiver back onto the cradle with an additional huff.

Agent #2 was calmly managing each passenger with a smile, apologizing for the delay and telling each one, "Let me see what I can do to get you on your way quickly." She clicked away at the computer and updated the passenger with each failed attempt, assuring them she had another option to try.

The biggest difference I saw was that the passengers in line #1 with the disgruntled agent were also disgruntled passengers, whereas the ones in line #2, while still just as much inconvenienced as the others, seemed calmer and more satisfied in the end.

It's interesting how the way we treat people matters.

In this stressful situation, it just made sense to smile and be kind to people. I read somewhere that people will generally mirror the attitude you give them. This was a perfect example of the truth of that statement.

A footnote: At 8:15 P.M. I had been waiting patiently a full nine hours. I was tired, bored, and hungry. Suddenly, a woman fainted and fell right in front of me. The paramedics were called and airport personnel scurried around her. I'm ashamed to say I found myself thinking, "Finally! Something interesting to help pass the time!" Does that make me a bad person?

Learning and Laughter

The Shock of Senior Status

The lady at the bank smiled as she looked over the paperwork for my new checking account. "You qualify for our free checking and free checks with our Senior Savers Account," she said as she continued to process the paperwork. What? Maybe I didn't hear her right.

"Is that for senior citizens?" I asked.

"Oh, yes," She replied. "We treat our seniors very well here at the bank."

I looked at her in disbelief. "I'm a senior citizen?"

She glanced down at the papers I had filled out, and said, "You're fifty-eight, so you qualify...."

"Wait a minute, are you serious?" I interrupted her.

She took a deep breath and said, "You're fifty-eight, right?"

Shocked and confused, I replied, "I am."

She continued moving papers around and clicking at the computer while she went on about the special things they do for seniors. I was in a fog. I should have known it was coming. Every day I wake up to find more of me has lowered. God's way of keeping us humble, I guess. I walked out to my car and took a good look at it—practical, reliable, and immaculate. Oh, Lord! I *am* a senior citizen!

All the way home, I wondered how my life would change now that I had graduated from middle age to senior status. However, once parked in the driveway, life took over. Four messages on my office phone had me putting out fires most of the afternoon. I had to get six customer orders to the post office, pick up the mail at the UPS store, drop off last-minute changes to the printer, and book my flight to Garden City for a business meeting. With that done, I quickly changed and ran off to meet Al Pylinski for dinner downtown. We've been great friends for over thirty years and never cease to find much to laugh about.

The menus arrived and we both pulled out our reading glasses. I informed him that we were senior citizens and told him what happened at the bank. Quickly our conversation became one laugh after another as we talked about getting older. We agreed the years were passing, but we didn't feel old. In fact, we both said we are enjoying life more now than ever. Life is one wonderful experience after another. Of course we will always treasure the time we had bringing up our children, but the freedom we have now is a welcome change.

What does it mean to be a senor citizen? It means independence, adventure, security, time, and I found out it also means you get discounts on almost everything. We both agreed this was an amazing time for us and we are grateful for the opportunities that lay ahead. Al suggested I may want to consider posing nude for the new Dove soap ads. I picked up my glass of red wine and as I clinked his glass I replied, "Great idea!"

The Laughter Pill

Whether you sell babushkas or Buicks, raise farm animals or children, perform brain surgery or stand-up comedy, stress is out to get you. We all know what it's like. We work from eight to five, rush to pick up the kids from day-care, take Johnny to soccer and Susie to dance lessons and have dinner on the table by six. Deadlines loom, restrictions stand in our way, due dates approach. Cars break down, babies cry, kids slam doors, cats pee on the rug, and dryers eat socks. We all face stressful situations every single day. The difference in how we live our lives is in how we handle what happens to us.

Stress is not an event; it is our reaction based on our perception of the event. The good news is that we are free to alter our perception. There is a better way to handle the craziness. How about just laughing that stress away? Laughter will lower your blood pressure and heart rate, elevate your mood, build confidence, promote teamwork, encourage problem-solving, prevent burnout, reduce fear, and even further promote good health.

Laughter helps us cope with what happens in our lives. Several years ago, I agreed to drop off my son at a halfway point so he could be a part of his father's family reunion. I called my former sister-in-law to get directions. As luck would have it, my ex-husband answered the phone. After twenty years of being my "ex" you would think he could handle giving me directions over the phone. Instead he called to his sister to do the chore, "Marie, it's the plaintiff." I am still referred to as the plaintiff? You have to learn to laugh at this kind of behavior or you can drive yourself crazy.

Was that any way to address the mother of his children? No. Was it funny? Yes, I believe it was. I justify it this way: if that were a scene on last night's situation comedy, I would have laughed. Almost everything that happens to us would be funny if it happened to someone else. We have to learn to see the absurdities in our everyday life and laugh them off. It really is a choice. Do I want to get stressed out over this or do I want to find the humor in it and laugh it off?

How we react to what happens in our day has to do with how we feel about ourselves. And how we feel about ourselves has everything to do with how we perceive a situation to be. Our perception of the situation, how we really see it, determines how we react to it. If we can change our perception, we can change our reaction, and in the end, change the results.

Let's take a look at how we get all stressed out in the first place. How do we get from happy-go-lucky children to nervous, frightened adults? Research from the *Book of American Averages* tells us that children laugh an average of four hundred times a day. By the time we reach adulthood, we reduce our laughter to only fifteen times a day. If laughter and humor is so important to our mental and physical health, then we had better find out how we got from a hardy four hundred to only fifteen laughs per day. We had better find out how we can get back to laughing our way to good health. By the time a child is only three years old he or she has heard "no" three hundred and fifty thousand times. "No!" "Put that down!" "Don't touch that!" "Stop it!" "No! No! No!" All this negativity...no wonder we stop laughing.

Think about when your children were babies, or being around babies in general. What is the first thing we all attempt to do when we pick up a tiny baby? If you said, "Make the baby laugh or smile," you are among the majority. We all make goofy faces and weird noises to try to get the baby to laugh or smile, and when the little one does, we praise. "Good baby!" The baby grows to be a cute little toddler and again we reinforce that laughter is good and right. When our toddlers do anything remotely funny, we laugh, and once again let it be known that we appreciate that wonderful sense of humor... until the child gets to be about eight or nine years old. Then when he or she starts to act silly we say, "What's so funny, young man?" "Wipe that silly smile off your face, little girl!" "You'd better straighten up and act like a lady." "Grow up." "You'll never be successful unless you get serious." "No one respects a wise guy!" "Quit acting so silly!!!" We are teaching our young people that in order to be successful, in order to gain the respect of our peer group, we had better be dead serious. I don't know about you, but I don't want to be anything that starts with dead.

We really need to look at and reassess the messages we are sending our children about laughter and humor. Our children's sense of humor will either blossom as they grow older or it will begin to wither away. Please don't let it wither away. They then become that horribly stiff person in the office who just can't have fun. This is the person who, to be politically correct, is "humor impaired"—too busy being important to laugh. It's the guy or gal who always has to rule the roost. The problem is that by ruling the roost all the time, we get stressed out, and all we end up doing is laying big fat eggs that everyone else in the roost has to clean up. The serious people in our lives are often seen as distant, negative, arrogant, or intimidating. Do you want others to read that from your face as you walk the office hallways? Is that what you want people to think of you when you push your cart down the aisle at the store? If you are not distant, negative, arrogant, or intimidating, then quit looking so serious. There was a time in my life when people would ask, "What's wrong?" and I would answer, "Nothing, why?" The response would always be the same, "You look mad." I wasn't mad, but I looked angry all the time. I was just preoccupied with worry and my face told the story. I think it is important to inform your face that you are happy, even while you have situations to take care of that may not be the most fun to have to handle. Try to play the part of a happy person on the outside and it will make a difference as to how you feel on the inside. Angels fly because they take themselves lightly. If you want to fly, lighten up.

Reintroduce yourself to your sense of humor. Be silly once in a while. Reconnect with the child in you. Find your joy. Your health depends on it. Start at home. Tuck a lottery ticket into your significant other's briefcase, pocket, or lunch bag. Take your granny to lunch for no reason. Buy flowers for a stranger. Mow your neighbor's lawn. Walk down a busy street and put quarters in parking meters that are about to expire. Fold someone else's laundry. It really is wonderful to do these things. It will put you in such a great mood. Take fun seriously. You can stop the world's worst day dead in its tracks by doing something just for the pure joy of it.

Remember, you can be as happy as you decide to be. If your life isn't what you think it should be, try to see it from a funny perspective.

> "I call my doctor up. Told him I had diarrhea.
> He put me on hold! Story of my life...no respect."
> —Rodney Dangerfield

Seven Cents

I have a confession to make. I love to find money. I will stop my car if I see something shiny and round on the pavement. I don't know if I can call this a hobby, a habit or an obsession, but I love to find money on the ground.

And I find it every time I go outside. My form of exercise is walking, but I can't just walk for the sake of taking a walk. I have to have a mission. My mission is: I don't come home until I've found some money. I usually find two or three pennies on a three-mile walk, but on a good day, a nickel or a dime may find its way into my pocket. I've found quarters on occasion, and one glorious day I found two five-dollar bills in the grass. I almost fainted. I also felt very sorry for the poor sap who dropped them. I walk with the intention of finding money. I actually go out my door and say I'm going to find money before I return.

This morning I was two miles into my walk and hadn't found a cent. I was getting discouraged and thought maybe today I wouldn't be so fortunate. I was about to give up when I had an attitude change. I thought about a speech I had to give on Saturday called "Developing Powerful Thinking." What a hypocrite I am! How can I teach others to think positive in order to create the life they want if I'm giving up so quickly? Immediately, right there in the parking lot of Bed, Bath and Beyond, I said to myself, Money comes to me. I find it everywhere. I'm finding money right now." In less than a second I saw a shiny object in front of me. WOW! A nickel! I picked it up and proudly put it in my pocket. I said out loud, Thank you Lord! and just as I did, I saw a shiny penny and then another. Amazing! Seven cents! It's like they simply fell from the sky just for me. That's seven cents I didn't have to work for. You have no idea how happy that simple gift made me feel this morning. Not the gift of seven cents—that was a bonus. The real gift was knowing that I have the power to intend good, positive things for me in my life. I have that power. Everyone does. What do you intend for yourself today?

Using Humor in Chronic, Autoimmune Disorders

April is National Humor Month, so do something silly. It's good for your health. Can your mental outlook really influence your health? Many experts say yes.

How much does the mind influence how the body functions? The question has prompted a great deal of debate in recent years as scientists have come to realize that mental stress has a negative effect on the immune system, while a positive attitude and a good, hard belly laugh benefits a person's health. As a matter of fact, laughter is one of the best antidotes for stress and anxiety.

I know firsthand the difficulty of living with chronic pain and depression. At twenty-three I was stricken with rheumatoid arthritis, and some days I hurt so bad I just want to curl up in a ball and cry. Instead, I fight my pain and depression with joy. I choose to find something to be happy about and engage myself in positive activities. When I get a flare-up and the pain is just too much to bear, I reach for my stash—my collection of laughter-filled videos and DVDs. *My Big Fat Greek Wedding, My Cousin Vinny,* and *Airplane* are my favorites. I also keep a collection of *I Love Lucy* reruns and the complete collection of *Seinfeld* handy. I know a hearty chuckle stretches the muscles from the diaphragm all the way to the scalp and releases the tension that causes fatigue, stress, and headaches, while giving me a giant burst of energy. Laughing releases endorphins, the body's natural pain killers and mood lifters.

We all go through difficult situations. Some manage to find a way to a better time and others whine and complain and share the misery with everyone. I say, "Pain is inevitable; the suffering part is optional." Living life in a joyful way is a choice we make every day. If you want to be happy—act happy. Bill Cosby said, "You can turn painful situations around through laughter. If you can find the humor in anything, you can survive it."

So the next time you have an ache or pain and you're feeling blue, don't whine and complain. Instead, find something filled with joy to do. Take a walk in the sunshine. Enjoy the changing of the leaves. Kiss your grandkids. Invite your funniest friend to lunch. Just don't sit there—do something silly!

Pray

Are you annoyed by rude, ungrateful people? What are they so angry about? When you are cut off on the highway or sassed by a store clerk, do you walk away cursing them under your breath or do you find yourself praying for God to bring them a tiny bit of joy? It makes sense to me that if you don't do anything to fix a problem, you may be part of the problem.

I've got a few people in my life who annoy me. They have bad attitudes. They complain about everything. They are rude. I pray for them all—even the ones I don't particularly like. I've been praying for the same souls for years with no visible change. Then lo and behold... miracles! Suddenly the angry neighbor is a joy to be around, the rude clerk actually gives me a smile, and the family member (who will go nameless) is actually grateful for something today. I could almost fall off my chair. What happened? When you pray for someone, you are wishing them well. I think simply sending good wishes their way day after day, month after month, and in some cases year after year, makes them able to feel that love and move out of their misery. It's just a theory. However it happened, my life is easier now that the people around me are happier. Their attitude toward life changed by receiving a friendly smile when they didn't deserve it, a reassuring hug after a barrage of complaints, or a consistent wish for happiness silently sent.

I thought, Hmm! If this works, we could change the world. So here's my plan: Join me in my quest to make this world a more joy-filled place. Join the "LaughterTude Club," a group of people with winning attitudes and a sense of humor. Members receive ideas and examples of how to live happier, healthier, more productive lives using humor as an antidote, and are reminded to Smile-It-Up instead of Stressing-It-Out. Members also have to meet a Giggle Quota, count their blessings, and pay it forward every single day in order to stay in the club.

It is my experience that generous, kind-hearted people are not only more successful in business, they are happier people and live longer than their cynical, serious sidekicks. It's not always easy to be kind or generous to mean-spirited people. My advice is to try it and see if you can change the attitude of others simply by being consistently kind, generous, and loving toward them. If you are willing to sign on for just six months, send me an email at smile

On your honor, you need to be kind, offer a smile or a helping hand, giggle every day, use your humor skills when stress comes your way, and be very grateful for what you have in your life. Oh, yes, and if you are so inclined, pray for joy for the people in your life who give you the most grief. I can't wait to see what happens in six months!

Influence

It was Sunday morning. The soothing voice of Charles Osgood offered a list of important people who died during 2009. He remembered how they made a difference in our lives by the way they lived.

As I listened to the stories and watched the faces of

scientists, movie stars, pop stars, and other legends fill the television screen, I thought not of those who have left this world, but of those who were born into it. Precious new lives were created this year. Miracle babies—216,000 of them—were born every single day into a world they know nothing about. I wondered what contributions they would make and how they would change this world. What would they become? How will they be influenced? Whose actions will motivate them, and whose beliefs will shape their minds?

Instantly, I had an Aha! moment. The massive responsibility we have as adults became almost overwhelming. Every single thing we do—each word we utter and every action we take—will be observed by the children in our lives. They will be affected by it. That made me want to be a better person immediately.

Sociologists tell us that even the most introverted person will influence 10,000 people in his or her lifetime. Some will be a good influence and others...not so much. I don't think we realize how important our actions, thoughts, and beliefs are, not just to our own children but to the little boy who sees us being rude in a store; to the child who plays quietly while his dad disrespects his mother; or to the little girl in a passing car who watches us toss a soda can out the window. Children are everywhere: in restaurants, shops, schools, churches, neighborhoods, and malls. They are little sponges, soaking up the influence we innocently offer them.

If we want to change this world for the better, we need to be very aware of how we influence those who will be running it in the future. Just a thought.

Kindness

Kindness is one of my favorite words. I remember seeing a sign in a secondhand shop that said KINDNESS PRACTICED

DAILY. It was no surprise to find that the lady that worked in that shop was sweet and kind. She made everyone who came into the shop feel welcomed. I am always drawn to people who are genuinely kind-hearted. I aspire to be known as a kind person. That's why I love the holiday season so much—kindness seems to be everywhere. People open the door for you, neighbors exchange cookies, we sing, we laugh, and all is merry. What happens to all that kindness once the tree is at the curb? We all know people who seem to put kindness away with the Christmas decorations. What can we do to change that?

The change begins with you and me. Kindness can and should be practiced every day and in every situation. Imagine how much better the world would be if everyone approached problems with decency, fairness, and civility. It is really such a simple concept, and yet being kind has an amazing power. When you make it a habit to use simple kindness in your everyday interactions, life is sure to be easier. Think about how you react to kindness. My grandmother, Rose Torsella, was a sweetheart. She never raised her voice. She moved with a gentle, elegant confidence and always had something pleasant to say. I would never have even thought of being anything but sweet to her. In fact, when I was with her, I was sure to be on my best behavior. It's common nature to treat someone in the same manner that they treat you.

It's a New Year and a time when we all attempt to make changes in our lives that lead us to be better as human beings. Try a little kindness this year and see if you don't end up with a kinder, gentler, more enjoyable time.

For the New Year, let's all resolve to practice simple kindness. As the old saying goes, "A spoonful of honey will catch more flies than a gallon of vinegar!"

I Can't Wait

If the stars should appear only one night a year, think how we would long for that special night! It would be astounding. Families would be out on the decks waiting with great anticipation. It would be such an event. Cameras would be set up to preserve the remembrance of such a spectacular sight. It would be an astonishing gift to be able to see such beauty. For most of us, the night sky glistening with stars is not so amazing. It's ordinary. We just expect it; take it for granted. There are plenty of nights to look at the stars. If we weren't blessed with this glorious gift each and every night, then when we *did* see a beautiful star, it wouldn't seem so ordinary. Our eyes would widen and our hearts would pound at the sight of a sparkling sky. It would be spectacular in our minds and hearts. And yet the stars are there every night; a magnificent gift for us to enjoy.

This speaks to a situation many of us experience: the giving of gifts to our grandchildren. Spectacular gifts. Gifts they expect. Gifts they take for granted. Why? Because, of course, for the same reason we take for granted all the gifts of the universe: plenty. When you are blessed with plenty, appreciation goes out the window.

We are guilty of burdening our family with plenty. Each time we enter a store, we exit with something for the kids. A new game or toy comes on the market and we get it for them right away. What would happen if they had to wait? If they didn't have a room full of toys at home, would any gift be exciting? Would one special gift given on a birthday be more amazing, more brilliant, if it weren't clouded by a plethora of others given every single day? What would happen if we stopped buying Xbox 360 gaming systems, PSP handheld games, *High School Musical* and *Baby Einstein* products? What if we didn't get her the Barbie three-story dream house complete with a stove that sizzles, a doorbell, house intercom, and a flushing toilet?

What if a child's birthday was simply a wonderful homemade cake with candles and a dining room full of family? What if all year long that child looked forward to the one day when he or she would be special? My birthday was important. I looked forward, counted the days, wished for that one special doll. Hopeful, but never knowing if I would be so blessed to have it. The anticipation was glorious. The day would come and my eyes widened and my heart pounded. It was special, out of the ordinary, amazing. My birthday would be an extraordinary event for me to enjoy just once a year. When it was over, I would spend another year anticipating that one spectacular day when I would be special again.

I am a grandmother to three great little boys. I have made a decision to give them glorious gifts. Gifts that will make their eyes widen and hearts pound. Gifts they will remember. I'm giving them time with me: time to bake, create, play, learn, read, and sing. But I won't be buying them the next best thing. The next best thing just won't be so special. Oh my stars, I can't wait!

Problems with the Well Endowed
(This fun essay was written when a good friend decided to get breast implants. Even after this warning she had them done anyway.)

Please read this warning before you make that important decision to live with bigger boobs.

Personally, big boobs are just a big pain in the...chest. You can't sleep well, because they're always in the way. It's like lying down on two rocks. At the theater, when you squeeze out of the seat to go to the bathroom, your left one always manages to hit the short, bald guy in front of you in the head. Your job options are limited. Forget about being a ballerina.

Never, ever try to eat a hot dog when you have big boobs, because mustard always drips. As a matter of fact, big boobs are the catch-all for food and drink. Women with flat chests never have spots on their shirts. The food just falls to the floor. With big boobs, your dry-cleaning bills are humongous. You should also know that once you lose a piece of jewelry down between your boobs, it just never can be found again. Hence the term "booby hatch."

Now, the one good thing is that if you're on your way to school and you're carrying a lot of things, and you just need an extra hand, a nice big boob can come in handy. Just lift one up and put all your pens and pencils underneath!

Another good thing is that you save money and time because you don't have to wear much make up. Once you have big boobs no man will ever look you in the eye again. They just say "Hello," and look right at your boobs. After that, they can't focus on anything else anyway; they're blinded somehow. I think it's called *boob blindness.* Okáy, I just wanted to get that straight before you take the plunge.

Out of the Mouths of Babes

Do you snap the minute something goes wrong? Are you the first to panic when you are pressed for time? Do you worry about things before they happen? And if they don't happen, do you wonder why? Maybe it's time to look for answers by spending some time with the children in your life.

Author Ashley Montagu says, "By learning to act more like a child, human beings can revolutionize their lives and become for the first time, perhaps, the kinds of creatures their heritage has prepared them to be—youthful all the days of their lives."

My niece Rae and her husband Garry were on their way back to New York after a family vacation in Disney World. All four of her children were securely buckled into their seat belts when the 747 they were on came into some very rough weather. The plane felt like it was jumping through the air. Rae looked around to find that many passengers were holding on for dear life. Panic, fear, and shock were prevalent throughout the cabin, when all of a sudden Rae's four kids all began to raise their hands up over their heads and shout in unison, "Weeeeeeeee! Weeeeeeee! Weeeeee!" The tiny tots giggled and continued to raise their arms over their heads each time the plane hit an air pocket. The children had decided to make the most of the situation they were in, while the adults in the cabin chose to be frightened. Rae said it was interesting to note that as soon as the passengers around her began to notice the children's reaction, they too began to laugh. She said the more people laughed the less stress there seemed to be in the cabin.

The truth is that we choose the reactions we have in life. The same thing was happening to both the children and the adults in the plane. They were all being rocked about due to the choppy weather conditions. The difference was that little Sara, Jacob, Natalie, and Makala decided to enjoy the ride.

This week when things start to get rocky, try thinking like a little child. What would your little niece or nephew, grandson or granddaughter do if they were in your shoes?

The next time you get together for a big family dinner, sit at the children's table. It's a lot more fun there.

Relax

With my office in my home, it's very hard to "get away from it all." There is always one more task that needs to be done, and relaxation is merely a nice idea.

One day, in an attempt to take better care of myself, I decided to have a little mini spa day and really treat myself to a quiet, soothing facial. (It's a trick I learned while stuck in an airport with nothing to read but one of those you-can-look-like-this-model magazines.) I put on a silk robe, lit a scented candle, and dimmed the lights. I whipped up some egg whites and mixed them with honey.

I pulled my hair back off my face and proceeded to lavish on the honey-and-egg concoction. Ooooh! It felt so good. Then I got my silk eye-beanie-bag-thingy out of the freezer and stretched back on the recliner. My new goose down quilt covered my body like a warm embrace. I placed the eye bag on my face and the coolness of the metal beans inside was a luscious gift against my tired lids. I proceeded to have the most relaxing forty-five minutes I have ever experienced...until the phone rang.

Since it was during working hours, I jumped out of the chair and raced to get the phone. I tried to pull the silk eye bag off my eyes as I ran, but the honey-and-egg mixture had glued it to my face. Afraid to pull my skin off, I left it in place and just Helen-Kellered my way to the phone and attempted to answer the call. All that came out was "mmmm mmmm mmmm." My mouth was also honey-glued shut. Panicked, I hung up the phone and ran to the kitchen sink to run warm water over my face in an attempt to loosen the mixture, which by now resembled sticky cement. As I came running out of the office I tripped over my briefcase and fell hard onto the carpet. My left cheek was now a bit rosier than my right one, but it matched the bruise on my arm so nicely. I was grateful for my tears as the warm, salty liquid helped to loosen the edges of my eye mask. The phone rang again. This time my priority was to get this sticky mess off my face. I decided this was a job for the sink sprayer. I didn't mind that water splashed all over the kitchen and me as long as the honey-and-egg mixture was finding its way down the drain. Finally, free from my face-mask prison, I went to the phone to check and see who my mystery caller was. Can you believe it was a Mary Kay Cosmetic lady who wanted to give me a free facial? I just absolutely cracked up.

Looser, Boozer, or Cruiser
I Have a Date
After the initial, "How are you?" "How's the kids?" and "How's the business going?" questions, my friends never fail to ask the dating question. "So how's your love life?" Each time I confess of the nonexistent love affair, I wonder why I don't try harder to find a man to love. Love seems to be all around me. Recently, I witnessed a bride and groom my own age madly in love with one another. Last week, I had dinner with two old friends who have been together happily married for forty-two years. This morning at the grocery store I ran into yet another happily married couple my age. Imagine it. Each time I see others in blissful love I wonder if it could ever really happen for me, and so I've put my toes back in the dating pool once again.

I met this man several months ago at a business meeting. He offered to help me with a sales program I was working to create. Over lunch, we talked about almost everything but the sales program. My first thought was, What a jerk! He just wanted to go out with me and used the sales program as an *excuse*. So I walked away from our perfectly pleasant lunch, never expecting or wanting to see him again. Men! They're so sneaky.

Since then, I've run into him several times, and each time he's polite, happy to see me, interested in my work, and greets me with a friendly kiss and hug. I'm very polite, but also very businesslike. Last night, I saw him again at a business dinner we were both invited to. He immediately greeted me with his warm smile, hug, and kiss. It felt normal to greet him this way, as if we were dear old friends or family. Again, he asked about my family, my work, and seemed genuinely interested. Remembering my quest to find real love and realizing I'll never find it unless I break out of my mold, I asked if I could sit at his table for dinner. This was a very big step for me. I was proud of myself. He was very gracious in making sure there was room for me and was a lovely dinner partner.

This morning I emailed him to thank him for making the evening enjoyable, and invited him to come hear me speak at a session I will be doing this week in Syracuse. He returned the email, saying he was going to try to make it, and then suggested we try to get together for a "cozy" dinner one night this week. He gave me his cell, home, and office numbers. I've decided to call him and make arrangements to go out to dinner. Enormous step.

I just hope I don't scare him off with my ridiculous inability to be myself in front of a man. I am typically judgmental and actually search for clues that he is a looser, a boozer, or a cruiser. In most cases, I really can't wait to go home. Looking back, I know that when I am alone with a man I turn into the most boring, shy, "I just want to go home and go to bed alone," type of girl. I'm working real hard to change my attitude. It's not easy. I'll keep you posted.

Common Sense Christianity

I was brought up a Catholic and went to Catholic schools. I married a Methodist. I liked the way they sang. Twenty years after I divorced him, I became a Methodist. But this isn't about religion. It's about living your life so that when it's time to turn to dust, you end up in a better place.

This is how I see things. I'm not a biblical scholar. In fact I often read passages in the Bible that I don't understand at all. There are so many Bible people all begotten and nobody's wearing protection. I do, however, find some passages in the Bible that are really meaningful to me. Those are the ones I read over and over whenever I need them.

Some people may get all up in arms over this essay, and say I don't know what I'm talking about. I don't claim to know anything about any particular religion. I don't claim to have all the answers, nor do I claim to understand all the messages in the Bible. I'm just offering you my view on the chance that it may help you in some small way.

When I write I will refer to Jesus as my Lord. I'm hoping people read this essay. Lots of different people. Whoever your God is, just think of Him or Her whenever I refer to My Lord Jesus. I believe that in order to get to heaven you just have to accept Jesus as your savior—that's it. Bingo! You're done. But in order to live your life the way He intended us to live, you need some good common sense.

Basic Idea: Be Nice to One Another

I have three sisters. I don't like everything about them. In fact there are some things about them that I totally disagree with. But I love my three sisters and I'm very grateful to have them in my life. I look at it this way: My

Lord gave me these three sisters as a gift. I love my Lord. I treasure all the gifts He gives me even if they are not the right size or the right color, even when they don't go with my décor. We do that don't we?

Imagine that your best friend in the world gives you a gift. It's something you would *never* buy for yourself. Since you love your friend, you keep the gift on the shelf forever, and each time you look at it, you think of your friend. Well, each time I look at my sisters—especially when they do or say something I may not agree with— I think of my friend who gave them to me and I just smile. This is the way I believe Jesus wants us to behave.

How do you check up on yourself to see how you are doing? How do you treat the people in your life? If you're a great friend but you're not on speaking terms with your sister, maybe you ought to think about how Jesus views that. If you are a wonderful co-worker, everyone at church loves you, and you do lots and lots of community service type things but you can't get along with your husband and nag him constantly, maybe you ought to think about how you look in the color red or how you would look with horns?

I don't mean that we have to be perfect little angels all the time. That's crazy. In fact, I can be quite mischievous myself at times, but I keep myself in check by asking myself what Jesus would think about the things I do and say and even the things I think about.

My friend Terri and I went to a garden party a few years ago. We come from big Italian families where food is the main event. This garden party was given by one of our petite, little, tiny girlfriends, and all she served was carrot sticks. We were starving. We were like rats looking for a scrap of cheese, and we were freezing to death because it was a very cool summer night. Terri and

I went into the house under the guise of having to use the bathroom. We went straight to the kitchen to see where the food was. We smelled nothing. Where was the food? It was supposed to be a barbecue. We saw a package of hotdogs defrosting on the counter and we were out of there.

Once in the car, we looked at one another and just cracked up. Where the heck were the cookies? The cheese? Where were the chips and the dip? What kind of party was that? We just cracked up because it was crazy to invite people over for hot dogs. In our family, we take extra napkins so we can take some cookies home for later. We wouldn't have had the strength to carry anything home from that party. We were starving. Terri and I laughed a lot in the car and really ripped that party apart. We went straight to the pizza parlor and had a wonderful meal and laughed some more. But we didn't hurt anyone. We would have never said anything to anyone else about that party. We love our little, skinny friend for who she is. She is a treasure, and we'll go to any party she has, but we'll eat a bowl of *pasta fagioli* before we get there and take a sandwich in our purse just in case we get hungry.

I think Jesus was up there laughing right along with us. He must have said to Saint Peter, "Watch this, I'm sending two little Italian girls to a party and there's no food. Watch them go nuts." He loves me. He loves Terri. And he loves our skinny, foodless friend.

Attitude Adjustment— Just What the Doctor Ordered

Olympic Gold Medalist Scott Hamilton said, "The only disability in life is a bad attitude." I agree. The good news is that we all have the privilege of deciding how we want to think. It's our choice. We can choose to be depressed and unhappy or choose to live life full of joy. The way you think, or your attitudes, are a direct result of the decisions you make.

I have rheumatoid arthritis. My worst enemy isn't the invasion of this painful disease on my body. My worst enemy is a bad attitude. The way that we allow ourselves to think has everything to do with how we feel. When I think about having RA, if I allow myself to entertain thoughts like, This is so unfair, Why me?, Bad things always happen to me, I'm so depressed, I ache all over, I hate this!, then my mind is filled with these negative thoughts, therefore, I'm giving it negative directions, resulting in a very bad attitude about my health. On the other hand, if I think—I am so grateful I am able to get up every morning and enjoy my life, I will do the very best that I am able to do, I know God loves me and is right beside me, I have purpose, I am committed to do all that I can to enjoy my life today and always, I am looking at all the beauty and goodness I have in my life, I'm looking forward to a great day, I am in good health, I love life—with these kinds of directions, I can't help but feel better and be happier.

As human beings, I think we are sort of programmed to look at the negative. That's why we have to work at staying happy. As soon as a bad thought comes into your mind, remove it. Have a mantra that you say whenever a bad thought enters the mind. Put a plan together before you get depressed and discouraged, and then when the nasty attitude hits, you'll be ready to attack! Here are some of my weapons against a bad attitude:

1. When I am asked how I am doing, my answer will be, "I'm doing terrific, how about you?" When you whine and complain to everyone you meet about how much pain you are in, it only fuels your mind with negative thoughts resulting in more pain!

2. I know that when I'm in pain, I get short-tempered and impatient. I will be sure to take a moment before I speak to people, take a deep breath, and treat people with the respect they deserve.
3. This pain will not last forever. I can get through this flare-up and I look forward to an easier day tomorrow.
4. Be real. It's not the end of the world. You're not going to die. It's pain. There are many people who have had to endure much worse. I can deal with this. I look at my entire world and not just a snippet of it. Basically, I've got a pretty good life and I'm grateful.
5. Write ten positive affirmations about your health. Post them on the fridge or in your office and repeat them anytime you start to hurt. "I understand that my body is fighting the effects of RA but I also know that I can choose to think of my grandchildren's smile; I can choose to walk in the garden and enjoy the flowers; I can choose how I think and I will. I am not a victim. I am victorious!

Remember, you are what you think about all day long. So think positive, happy thoughts.

Advent

Growing up in a strong Italian Catholic family, I was taught to respect my elders. That meant that I did whatever was expected of me—no questions asked. Each time I entered a church, I automatically genuflected and made the sign of the cross. During mass, I responded in perfect Latin. I knew my prayers by heart but was never very clear what they meant or why I did the things I did. I only knew that it was expected and so I did it.

Advent simply meant Christmas was coming. It meant

the soft glow of candles, gaily decorated presents, the joyous color red and *more*. There was more of everything during that time—more shopping, cooking, and cleaning. We had to make sure everything was spotless and festive. Dad made sure the beautiful lights were hung on the house and Mom got all those treasures out of the cellar to put on display. It's when we used our best china and silver and wore our very best clothes. We had to get ready for all the relatives and friends that came to visit us at this time. For me, Advent had always been a time to get ready for visits from the people we loved.

My spiritual life changed in 1971 when I came to a tiny Methodist church in Edmeston, New York. It was there that I left behind the ceremonial rituals I had come to know and embraced the everlasting love of Jesus.

Advent to me is a celebration of His promise. Christ was born and Christ will come again. Now I know that the Advent season is a time to remember how fortunate I am that He came. It is a time to prepare myself for the coming of Jesus at Christmas. The Advent season is a time when I look at the way I live my life and remind myself to live the way Jesus wants me to. He is coming and I want to be ready. It is a time of giving and of sharing our attitudes of Faith, Hope, and Love. That is the spirit of the season of Advent.

When I was a little girl we worked to prepare our house for the coming of our loved ones. We wanted to be ready when they came. Now I know that Jesus is coming to my house, and I want to be ready when He comes.

I know that the Lord loves me and that He will always be there for me. I know that He watches over me and knows what is right for me. He must have wanted me to have the joy of slowing down and reflecting on this season. I think that is why He inspired me to write about Advent.

No matter what your religious or ethnic background is—take a moment by slowing down and reflecting on what the season of Advent really means to you.

The Long Walk to Christianity

We were supposed to be "in prayer," but after the second time my fingers slid over the wooden rosaries, I was bored. Saint Cyril's Academy for Girls was a Catholic boarding school in Pennsylvania where most Saturdays were spent in complete silence and prayer. I was sent there because I was a problem child. This place was intended to straighten me out. In a way, it did. It is where I first became interested in theology. Forced to repeat prayers over and over and to attend Latin mass every day seemed meaningless to me. The repetitive acts left me yearning for something more. Asking too many questions in our daily religion classes, I became the problem child at the academy. Sr. Mary Gerard told me to just accept things and stop asking so many questions. When I told her I'd like to become a nun after graduation she told me I'd "make a better mother than a nun." I was expelled for bad behavior.

The curiosity didn't stop. Something about this religion phenomenon was calling me, tugging at me. Wanting to know the truth, I church-shopped. After several stops at Catholic, Baptist, Lutheran, and Episcopal churches, I found a home in a tiny, small-town Methodist church. They were desperate for young people who were willing to work. Becoming a children's Bible schoolteacher was a great way for me to learn along with the kids. It was there that I started to actually read the Bible. The more I read, the more I wanted to understand. My constant questions were getting answered. Although I felt I was closer to Jesus, I still felt that I was missing something big. I started to investigate by reading whatever I could find, watching TV evangelists, and sneaking over to a Pentecostal church every now and then. I was fascinated at how involved some people were. They raised their hands, closed their eyes, cried real tears, and shouted hallelujah! I watched nervously as some lay down in the middle of the aisle, mumbling to some invisible force. Weird. But they all loved Jesus. I wanted to love Him, too. I always believe He lived, He was the Son of God, He was powerful, but I didn't really understand how to love Him.

It has taken me thirty years to really love the Lord Jesus with all my heart. This means that I accept the teachings of the apostles, that I know Christ's death washed away my sin and disabled death itself. This is Christianity. What greater love could there be? He died for me. I wasn't there. I didn't see Him. I never touched His robe. But I know He lived because I believe it on authority. That is what faith is. If I only believe what I personally see, think of what a small world I would have. I believe that God loves me not because I'm a good person, but rather His love is why I want to be a good person, good mother, good neighbor, and good citizen. I believe that in order to be forgiven, I must forgive others even though that can be difficult at times. I believe in daily prayer, reading the Bible, and attending church service, because as a Christian I need to be reminded. I think we need to be reminded more than educated about God's love. We all know right from wrong no matter what our religion or faith is. By attending services, I am reminded of what Christ did for me. That makes me want to be a better person for Him. Finding the true love of Jesus is like suddenly becoming aware of everything that is good. I am awake now and all that I have and do and all that I am was given to me by His love. I thank Him every day, all day long for everything. I thank Him for my home, my children, and my work. I thank Him for a good cup of coffee in the morning. I thank Him for a car that runs.

Some may say it is hard to be a Christian, but I think the opposite is true. I have a constant companion who is always right here with me, picking me up when I fall, reminding me not to worry and stress over things I can't change, offering me hope when things are difficult, and loving me not because I'm perfect but just because I'm me.

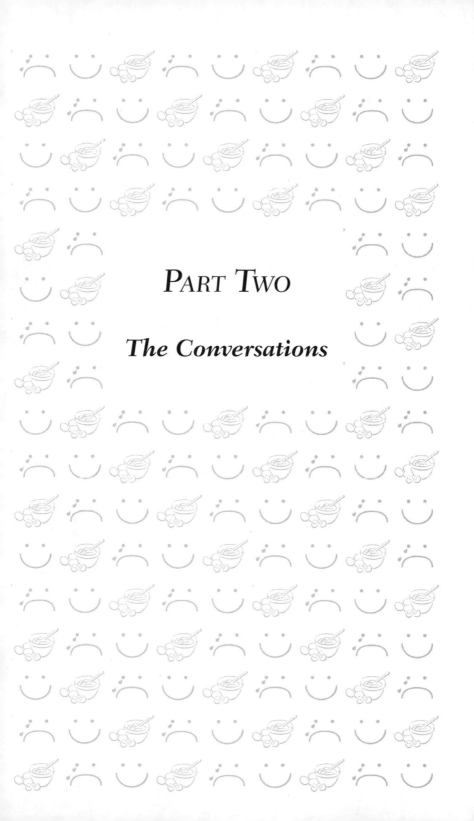

PART TWO

The Conversations

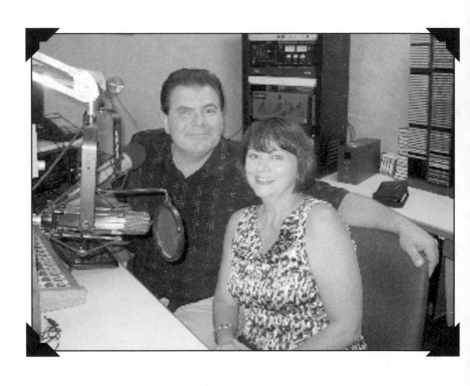

Every Wednesday morning, I am fortunate to be able to offer funny stories, interesting ideas, and life lessons to the listeners of Central New York radio. On *The Gary Dunes Morning Show* on WSEN 92.1 FM, Gary and I talk about life. Whatever is happening in our lives ends up on the radio: the silly stuff, things that make us mad, things that bring us joy, and the lessons we learn. Over the years, fans have asked if there was a way to get copies of those conversations. We believe in "ask and you shall receive." The following are conversations between Gary and me on the air, exactly as they occurred. The grammar may not be correct, but I wanted you to read what we talk about.

The Power of Laughter

GARY: I've been to conferences where you've been the speaker and there is a very funny side to what you do and you have people laughing, cracking up, really enjoying everything, but there is also a serious side to it, too, isn't there?

YVONNE: Yes, because the whole point is teaching people how to use humor to get through the difficulties in life. A woman came up to me after a presentation and she talked to me about the loss of her husband. She said, "My husband died last year and I cried non-stop for weeks. I was

making myself sick, I cried so much. My heart was broken. He was my soul mate, my love for over forty years,
and I didn't know how to live without him. My sister-in-
law invited me to go to the Bahamas. She thought the
change of pace would do me good. And it did. I stopped
crying and tried to enjoy the few days in the sun. The
last night of the vacation I was sitting in a crowded restaurant, everyone was having a great time, the music was
beautiful, the view of the ocean was lovely, the food was
delicious and I thought...my husband would have just
loved this." At that moment, she burst into uncontrollable tears. You know, the ugly cry....

GARY: Sure.

YVONNE: ...and people stopped talking and looked over at
her. Then the waitress came to the table with the check
and she sort of froze, and her sister-in-law looked up
at the waitress and said, "She does this every time the
check comes." And she said, "At that moment, I burst
into laughter. And it was uncontrollable laughter."

That is the positive power of humor. When it can take
you from a moment of deep sadness and pain and take
you to a place of joy in an instant. That's why this is so
important. Because it helps us get through the difficulties that life hands us. It doesn't cure you or bring back
your lost love, but it will get you through the moment
and sometimes that's all we really need.

From a Child's Perspective

GARY: Last week I had the opportunity to attend a lun-
cheon where you were the keynote speaker and you told
a lot of funny stories about your family. How about sharing one with us?

YVONNE: I am so blessed with this very large and extremely colorful extended family, and one of my sisters is always calling with a silly story for me. This week my sister Donnarae was enjoying dinner with her husband and four grandchildren when she said to her husband, "Mary and Chuck are leaving for Florida this week." Immediately her little granddaughter Sarah dropped her fork and looked up wide-eyed, and said, "Who's Chuck?" My sister said, "Chuck is Mary's husband. Why?" Little Sarah pushed herself away from the table and folded her arms and said, "So Mary has a husband *and* a little lamb?"

It was hysterical, but you know our kids are wonderful little humorous beings. They are filled with silly gems because they are so innocent and pure. Little kids don't panic about getting places on time. They don't worry about things before they happen. They don't stress out about how they look or what they are eating. If you find yourself full or stress and worry, it may be time to spend some time with the children in your life.

Author Ashley Montagu says, "By learning to act and think more like a child, human beings can revolutionize their lives and become for the first time, perhaps, the kinds of creatures their heritage has prepared them to be—youthful all the days of their lives."

Home Depot Humor

GARY: So you bought a shed recently. Tell me all about that.

YVONNE: I did. I had a very good experience at the Home Depot. I went in there to buy a shed. And I don't know anything about sheds, Gary, I know about shoes!

GARY: Okay, I hear ya.

YVONNE: So I had to ask a million questions. I decided on this particular shed but still I had to ask more questions about how it goes together and I realized men were piling up behind me with lumber and sheet rock. They were getting impatient with all my questions.

There were three men all waiting to talk with the clerk that was finishing up my paperwork. They were shifting their weight from one foot to the other, taking deep breaths...all the signs of being impatient...in a hurry... frustrated with me for asking so many questions about the shed before buying it. They were anxious to get their purchases and get on to work, I'm sure. But this is a perfect example of using your comic vision to kind of change the mood in any situation. Right then everyone was stressed out.

Next to the counter was a coffee pot and cups. All of a sudden, the man that was waiting next to me looked at the free coffee and then looked over at me and said in a sort of sexy way, "So...can I buy you a cup of coffee?" The three guys behind us laughed, I laughed, and the clerk laughed, and then he poured me a cup of coffee. It was just something silly he thought of to do and it totally relieved everyone's stress. That is a perfect example of using your comic vision to turn an unpleasant moment into a pleasant one. So use your comic vision at work, in the car, with the kids, with the spouse, in the store or wherever you happen to be.

Halloween

GARY: Halloween is just around the corner any plans you have for Halloween?

YVONNE: Gary, I dress up. Every Halloween. I have a gypsy outfit that I wear with the boots and the whole bit, and I dress up.

GARY: To answer the door?

YVONNE: Yep. For the kids. I love the little kids.

GARY: Very cool.

YVONNE: This is actually a great time to find out a little bit more about your own children.

GARY: How so?

YVONNE: You ask your kids, not just what do you want to be for Halloween, but what would you be if you could be anyone or anything in this world or even beyond. If I had a magic wand and you could be anything you want, what would it be? It's interesting what they say. Their answers kind of help you figure out what your kids are thinking about...

GARY: Sure

YVONNE: ...who their heroes are, you know, who they look up to or in my case...which chores they are opposed to be doing.

GARY: What do you mean by chores?

YVONNE: When my son Johnny was about four, he was in a talent/beauty contest and the host asked him what would he like to be when he grows up, and Johnny looked right at her and said, "I would love to be a road!"

GARY: A road?

YVONNE: Yep, he said, "I want to be a road." The host was so shaken by his answer that she just moved on to the next kid. When I got him in the car, I asked him why he wanted to be a road, and he said, "Oh, Mom, it would be so great to be able to play with my trucks and cars all the time, and if I were a road I would never have to pick them up and put them away." That's the way a four-year-old thinks. That's a conversation I would never have had with my son if he hadn't been asked that question. I think it's a great time of the year to ask your kids, "What would you like to be if you could be anything at all?" and it really helps you to understand what they are thinking about.

GARY: Great idea Yvonne.

I'm Stressed

GARY: Stressful times are upon everybody these days with the price of gas and the financial situation. What's your advice on dealing with stress?

YVONNE: We all know stress is not good for us. I read recently that the symptoms of too much stress in our life is excessive eating, excessive drinking, not getting enough exercise, and overspending, which scared me because that's my description of a great day. If I can have a delicious meal, a good glass of wine, skip the gym, and buy three pair of shoes that I don't need—I'm happy. So that kind of scared me when I read that. But I guess if you do that to excess then you have to think about better ways to reduce the stress. When I do find myself worrying about something or getting stressed out, I consciously make a decision to do something fun. I force myself to get out of the house and meet up with some funny friends or I pop in a laughter-filled video—that tells you how old I am because they're not DVDs they're videos. *Throw Mama from the Train, My Cousin Vinny, and My Big Fat Greek Wedding* are some of my favorites. Anything that will get me laughing out loud helps me to reduce my stress.

We know laughter is good for your health and well-being. I mean, Joan Rivers is alive and Dr. Atkins is dead! That's proof enough for me. If you think about the people in your own life who find a way to laugh a lot, in most cases they are not the same ones who get stressed out and worry a lot. They may have the same types of problems and situations in life that the stressed-out people do, but they find a way to look at life differently. It's really all about your perception—the way you look at what is happening to you.

Laughter won't change the situations in your life, but laughter may help you to see and react to it differently. Changing your perception can change the outcome of any situation.

GARY: I find myself buying box sets: *Everybody Loves Raymond, The King of Queens, Two and a Half Men.* And I pop them in whenever I need a little jolt.

YVONNE: That's a perfect thing to do. I have every Seinfeld episode. They just make me laugh. It just changes your perception and you are able to attack whatever is your stress point in a more effective way.

Travel

GARY: I know you travel a lot, Yvonne, and that's got to be a pain, isn't it?

YVONNE: Well, for me, I find a way to get through the difficulties of travel. But I'm telling you, people complain about travel all the time. Everyone had "the worst flight ever!" No—if you had the *worst flight ever* you won't be here to tell about it right?

GARY: That's right yep.

YVONNE: I figure if the guy lands the plane and I get to get off, that was a good flight. I fly to a different city nearly every week and I never leave home without my humor tools. It's about having fun, seeing the humor where others miss it. Why are people so surprised when the airlines lose your luggage? They are going to lose your luggage; just expect it. Or do something about it. Take action.

Honestly, I've been flying now for fourteen years and I have never lost my luggage. You know you're waiting in that black circle of doom. People are praying their black bag with a piece of red string comes out the shoot. I know mine will arrive. Mine is different. I keep one of those fake hands with the shirt attached coming out the top. Nobody ever touches my bag.

Humor is all around us. We just don't see it because we are always thinking about something else. Everyone is on the cell phone or checking their Blackberry—are they all really that important that they can't just relax for an hour? Everyone complains that they are tired and have no time and then the airlines give us two hours to just sit and be still, and instead, we use that time to stir up negative emotions. The minute a flight gets delayed or we get stuck on the tarmac, the phones come out. People cannot wait to share their misery. I choose to have fun no matter where I go, and you can't stop me. My mom used to tell me constantly to act like a lady, but really, I find it's much more fun to act like a little kid. That way, you see all that humor other people miss. People-watching is a great pastime. I do it all the time at airports. You can always find people doing really funny things.

GARY: Makes the time go by fast

Discipline

GARY: Well I guess congratulations are in order. Your daughter had another little baby.

YVONNE: She did. She had another little boy. We named him Jack. He's as cute as he can be, you know. She has a two-year-old, Joey, and he's into everything. You know how two-year-olds are. She also has a stepson, Christian, who is ten. So she has her hands full. And I talk a lot about discipline with my daughter because today's discipline is very different from when I was a kid. When we were kids, if you did something wrong, your dad would give you a little whack, you know.

GARY: Yep. That's the way it was.

YVONNE: Not hard, just a little whack on the side of the head...with his belt...or a metal buckle. You'd bleed a little, get a Band-Aid, but you never did that thing again. You learned. Right?

GARY: That's right.

YVONNE: But now we don't hit our kids. We give them time-out. Time-out doesn't work. That's what happened to the Menendez brothers. They sat in their rooms thinking, We have to get rid of her! I'm not saying we should hit our kids. I'm just kidding and teasing, but I don't think sending them to their rooms—which, by the way, is like sending them to an amusement park now—I don't think that works. They love going to their rooms. They're full of toys, video games, and computers. I think the best thing to do is teach them that every action has a consequence. If they throw a truck at their little brother then they lose the truck. It stays on top of the fridge for a week. I give young mothers today a lot of credit, because it is not easy.

Holiday Gratitude Chain

GARY: Thanksgiving is upon us and I plan to eat a lot and often.

YVONNE: I do, too. It actually is my favorite holiday, because I love to cook, I love to bake, and I love to eat!

GARY: Our whole family gets together. It's a big family thing for us over at my sister's house with her kids.

YVONNE: I normally have it at my house, but my daughter said, "Gee, Mom, you've been traveling so much, how about I have Thanksgiving at my house?" I thought, Oh, isn't that sweet of her! and then she says, "But you need to make all the pies and could you make your *pasticiotti* and your casseroles?" So I've got a whole list of things I have to make and cart over to her house. What's the point? The only thing she's doing is the turkey.

GARY: She should have brought it to your house.

YVONNE: Exactly. But we will have a good time no matter where we are. I've got a great idea for my three grandsons for Thanksgiving Day. We are going to make a holiday gratitude chain. You know how little kids are always asking how many days till Christmas or Hanukkah?

GARY: Great idea.

YVONNE: Well, you have them make a chain out of construction paper with 27 links, one for each day between Thanksgiving Day and Christmas Eve. This gives the kids something to do on Thanksgiving while the turkey is in the oven. Mom cuts strips of construction paper ahead of time and all the kids need are some crayons and a stapler or tape. But here's the good part: You ask the kids to write something they are grateful for on each ring of the chain. Like, "I'm grateful for my dog," "My mom," "I don't have to do dishes," "Don't have to go to school today."

GARY: Nice.

YVONNE: Then, each night before they go to bed, they remove one link of the chain till no more are left, and presto! It's Christmas Eve.

GARY: sounds good. Well you have a great Thanksgiving and I'm going to try not to eat so much.

Time to Relax

GARY: I tried to get a hold of you a few times last week. You've been on the road working a lot lately.

YVONNE: Yep, in one week I worked in Milwaukee, Detroit, Cleveland, and Vegas—all in one week

GARY: That sounds like the song: Detroit, New York City—James Brown song

YVONNE: Exactly, except for I didn't have as much fun as *he* probably did. It was a long week, Gary. In Vegas, I worked for Xerox Women's Alliance, and we had 700 high-powered women executives there. One young woman shared an interesting story with me. She had two young children and was a busy working mom. She was out raking leaves with her kids and she got a great big pile all neatly stacked and went to get a plastic bag to put them in.

When she got back, her kids were running headfirst into the nice, neat pile of leaves, and they were laughing and screaming and having fun like kids do. Immediately, she yelled, "Get out of the leaves right now. You're messing up the leaves." And her littlest one popped her head up out of the pile and said, "Geez, Mom, we were just having fun."

GARY: Awwwww.

YVONNE: She said, "I took a deep breath and thought, FUN! When was the last time I actually had any fun?" You know, because she's so busy, and every mother is like that. It doesn't matter where you work. Even a stay-at-home mom. You've got so many things going on, you forget to make time to relax and just have some fun once in a while. She put down the bag, the rake, and dived headfirst into the pile of leaves with the kids. She said, "You should have seen the look on the kids' faces. They acted like Christmas morning. They were so happy." She realized one of the best gifts we can give our kids is to relax and have some good old-fashioned fun with them. I know we can get frazzled trying to get chores done, but try to remember to take a deep breath, relax and have fun—that's the key.

Calm down

GARY: I don't know. Is it just me or the time of year? But everyone seems to be overloaded, rushing around. Everything's hustle and bustle. Is it just me or...?

YVONNE: No, it's everybody, and I'm just like everyone else. I tend to run like a chicken with its head cut off, especially at this time of year. I learned a good lesson this week, Gary: You can really mess up when you rush. I'm having some work done at the house. I decided to put a new bathtub in, have my ceilings painted, and upgrade my closets. So I called a bunch of people to get quotes. One lady answered the phone and said, "Steve usually does the quotes, but he won't be able to call you today. His mother is very sick." So I said, "Okay, no rush. Hope everything is okay." Then I left messages with several other companies to give me quotes. Later that afternoon I get a call. The guy says, "This is Steve. You called about your closets?" I said, "First of all, Steve, how's your mother?" He kind of hesitated, and then he said, "My mother? She's passed away."

GARY: Oh, boy.

YVONNE: I said, "Oh, my goodness, I'm so sorry." He said, "Do I know you?" Now, I'm thinking he recognizes my name from hearing me speak somewhere or, the radio, so I said, "I'm not sure. You might." He sort of hesitates and then sets up an appointment for the next day. I'm like, "Aren't you going to be busy tomorrow?" I'm thinking his mother just dropped dead, right?

GARY: Sure, yes.

YVONNE: He says, "Lady, I got nothing better to do tomorrow than fix your closet." I'm like, okay, back up this truck. I said, "I was told you wouldn't be calling me today because your mother was sick." He says, "Honey, you got the wrong guy. My mother died in 1982."

GARY: Wow.

YVONNE: I realized I must have mixed him up with a different Steve, right? I told him what happened and we had a little laugh about it. Really, all my rushing around trying to do three things at once and all the bits of papers I have on the desk just messed me up. I totally confused this guy with one of the other workmen. We had a good laugh over the confusion, but the lesson is: Slow down, take a breath, do one thing at a time, and life will be a lot easier.

Love Gift Box

GARY: Yvonne, I know you are a keynote speaker, but you're an author, too. You've published several books and one of them, *Bits of Joy*, has one hundred and fifty positive things to do, and one section talks about things to do with your children. Can you share an idea with us?

YVONNE: Okay, well, actually, this is a good time to talk about generosity, because of the holidays.

GARY: Sure.

Yvonne: I've got a great idea that teaches your children about being generous. Kids learn best by our example, so we need to be mindful of how we act and the things we do, because kids learn by watching us. When my kids were little, I really didn't have a lot of money, but we used to have what I called the "Love Gift Box" and it sat right in our living room on the TV set—you keep it in a prominent place in your home and get your family members to drop spare change each evening into the box. The kids see you doing it and you encourage them to do it as well. Tell the kids the love box money is to do something generous and kind for someone else. They see the money pile up. You are teaching your kids how to save and you can make it a family project to sort of research what to do with the money. It may be something simple, like, you go buy some groceries and take them to a shelter, or use it to buy ingredients and make cookies for a neighbor.

Gary: Oh, nice, yes.

Yvonne: You have to use the money to do something nice for someone else. Buy a plant for a neighbor. It teaches the kids that it's not all about, "What am I gonna get?" It's about giving. It teaches the kids how wonderful it feels to be able to give. I do something a little different with my grandson. I give him five dollars a week allowance and he has to give the first dollar to charity, the second dollar he puts into savings, and he has the remaining three dollars to do whatever he wants with. He said, Nonni, "It's not really allowance because I don't have to do anything to get it." What he doesn't realize is that the lessons he is learning about saving and generosity are priceless. I think it's important to teach your kids that it's not all about receiving. It's about giving back—great lesson.

Family Tradition

GARY: Christmas is right around the corner. So many people have so many different traditions, different nationalities, and stuff. What are some of your traditions? Share them with us today.

YVONNE: Well I'm full-blooded Italian, Gary. We get together on Christmas Eve, do you?

GARY: Absolutely.

YVONNE: We used to do the traditional twelve-course fish dinner at midnight. A fish for every one of the apostles. I think that's why we did it. I don't even know!

GARY: Yes, I think that's it.

YVONNE: I remember when I was a kid, there were just bowls of fish all over the kitchen. Our house smelled like a fish market. We still celebrate on Christmas Eve. After my father passed away, it seemed like every year we lose a fish. But that's the thing about traditions. As your family grows or gets smaller, your traditions may change, and that's fine. I think the problems occur when people try to keep things "the same way it always was," and then they get disappointed because it doesn't work out the way they expected it to.

GARY: Oh, yes, you're right.

YVONNE: The best thing to do is just remember to enjoy your family and have a good time together. We do a number of things. Since my father passed away, the first year I got clown noses for everyone in the family, and I said, "You don't come in unless you wear the clown nose." We wanted to do something different to sort of get us through, and so we all wore red sponge clown noses all through the night. We wore them while we ate, opening the presents, singing the Christmas carols. My mother made us take them off to go to midnight mass, but other than that, we had them on all night, and it really got us laughing, because you just look at someone with a clown nose on and you have to laugh because they look so funny. It really helped us change the way we were feeling, especially that one Christmas right after my father passed away. Now, my sister Donnarae is in charge of bringing something funny for us each year. She introduced us to the giant feet we had to wear one year and the head boppers—just anything silly. It really adds to the joyfulness that this season is really all about. And it's a way to get everyone to join in the fun. Now it's a tradition with us.

I bake a birthday cake on Christmas Eve and have the little kids sing happy birthday to Jesus and blow out the candles so that they can understand the real reason for the season. It gets kind of out of hand. It's so commercialized.

GARY: Yes, it is.

YVONNE: And we can't help that. I think it's important to be sure the kids understand what the holiday is about. That's why we have the birthday cake. The thing to do is introduce a tradition that you can keep in your family. Make it special. Something you look forward to.

GARY: Well, I'm gonna have some calamari tonight, some haddock, and some shrimp.

YVONNE: Oh, you still do all the fish?

GARY: We do all the fish with my family. I'm really looking forward to it.

New Year's Resolution

GARY: Now, I'm off today but I had to come in special to wish my good friend Yvonne a Happy New Year. Here we are another New Year's Eve and another year gone by. What's your New Year's resolution?

YVONNE: Gary, I don't do New Year's resolutions.

GARY: I don't, either. A lot of people do, though, right?

YVONNE: A lot of people do, but I don't do resolutions anymore, because, let's face it, I don't know about you, but I never keep them, and then I feel like a big loser, so I don't do that.

What I like to do every New Year's Eve before I go to any party or anything is sit down and make a list of all the things I've accomplished in the past year. And it could be simple things or it could be big deals—it doesn't matter, but whatever you think you accomplished in the year, you make a note of it. It could be work-related, family, health, financial, vacation, spiritual goals, whatever it might be. Once you get thinking about it, you end up with a nice list of accomplishments and you feel good about yourself. It's a great way to keep track. I write down every book I read so I can say, "Wow! I read twenty-two books this year." It could be: I put a new garden in, I painted the garage. You know, things like that. Whatever it may be that you accomplished. I redecorated the living room or simple things like I got my Christmas lights up before the snow hit. Instead of saying, "Oh, man, I messed up. I didn't keep the resolution," you look at the list and you say, "Wow! In this year I accomplished this. Not bad." You're not gonna believe what I put on my list this year.

GARY: What's that?

Yvonne: I went back to my natural hair color. I looked like an idiot with this blond hair. What kind of Italian has blond hair? What was I thinking? My eyebrows are jet black, for Pete's sake! So I feel better about that, and that went on the list. Somehow looking at your successes puts you in a better place to begin the New Year.

Attitude

Gary: With the economy what it is, and people worried about jobs, what kind of advice do you have for keeping a joyful outlook?

Yvonne: You know, Gary, it's really a choice you make to keep looking at life from a joyful perspective, no matter what is going on. No matter how bad the day is going—to be able to find something to laugh about. It almost becomes a way of life. My sister Donna is a great example of someone who always finds something to laugh about. She was having a rough day last week and nothing was going her way. She was really getting frustrated and decided to stop at a Dunkin Donuts and take a break. She walked in and there was a long line, which just added to her frustration. When she finally got to the counter with my eighty-four-year-old mother beside her, she said loudly, "Give me two scotch and sodas on the rocks!" She just has that funny sense of humor and is not afraid to do silly things at the drop of a hat. She said just seeing the look on the kid's face behind the counter got her laughing. Soon the rest of the people in the shop were all laughing and commenting about what she said.

Being able to laugh when your day isn't going as planned sort of gives you a break—an opportunity to take a breath and look at things from a new perspective. The power of humor, being joyful, is really a choice we make. Yes, we all have to tighten our belts right now and things may not be perfect. Take a break, look around you, and I promise you will find something to smile about.

Sunday Dinner

GARY: I know a lot of people with an Italian background who used to have dinner on Sunday with the family. I know we always used to do that growing up with my grandparents and stuff. Do you still do that?

YVONNE: Well, you know, we do our very best to try to keep that tradition going. Having dinner with the family on Sunday has always been part of my heritage and my life growing up, just like you. We do try to do it, but it's not always easy. My son-in-law works full time and goes to school some nights and with three kids, someone always has to be somewhere, karate class, ball practice. It's always something. We try to get together. I look forward to fresh bread, sauce and meatballs, the smell, the way the table looks, it's all part of my heritage. I want to be sure my kids and grandkids enjoy that as well. It's something we can count on every Sunday. Dinner with the family. That is where you really bond with each other and create some wonderful memories. As a matter of fact, this past Sunday I had the kids over and my daughter Aubry was telling a story and she spelled out a cuss word instead of saying it. My eleven-year-old grandson Christian says, "Hey, some kids can hear spelling you know!"

Later, when someone used bad manners at the table he said, "Don't you know how to use your ediquit!" And we were like, ediquit? What the heck is ediquit?

It ends up being a laughfest for us most Sundays, and that is a great way to sort of relax and put all your concerns on a shelf for one day in the week and just enjoy the family.

When I was a little girl, we ate dinner in the dining

room every Sunday. We used the good china and silver
and a linen tablecloth. We had our Sunday dinner together. You don't have to use china and linen, but for me,
I like to keep the tradition going.

GARY: I used to love that growing up.

YVONNE: It was a special tradition that brought us together
as a family. With everyone so busy these days it's important to find time to connect. Start a tradition with your
family. Share a special meal. Bring your family together
around your dining room table.

Laughing at Work

GARY: Yvonne you work with some big corporations. How
do you get the bosses to hire you to teach them how to
laugh at work?

YVONNE: You wouldn't think they'd want me to do that.
Truth is, I have more respect for a person who is flexible
and can have a laugh every now and then. I worry about
people who think they have to be so serious all the time.
Wouldn't you rather do business with someone who can
make you laugh? Or who can laugh at himself?

GARY: Absolutely

YVONNE: I know I would.

GARY: I know going to a restaurant, I want a guy that's
friendly—the bartender or the waitress—that's very
friendly, someone that makes you feel good.

YVONNE: Exactly. People who can find humor in difficult
situations are able to reduce the stress level, which makes
it a lot easier to solve problems. I'd rather be spending
my leisure time with someone who can find the silly side
of life as well. I was walking into a mall one time with

my friend Tonja. She's from Nashville. We passed this kid
with dreadlocks—long, thick, twisted hair. She looked at
him and then said, "You know, I washed a rug one time,
come out the dryer looking like that." Some people can
just see humor everywhere and make you laugh. That's
the kind of person you want to be around—someone
that can make you laugh and put all your troubles on
hold for a few minutes. I think it's important to be flexible and to be able to see the funny side of life at work
and at home.

Funerals and Elastic

GARY: Where have you been working? You been around
home? I see your car in the drive. I never know if your
home or up in the air somewhere.

YVONNE: Actually, I've been blessed to have a bit of local
work. In fact, just recently I worked for Time Warner here
in Syracuse and I got a great funeral story from Chris,
one of the folks at the conference. That's the best part of
my job, when people come up and share a funny story
with me.

Chris said she was at a funeral with her friend Marie
and they were standing right next to the family of the deceased. Marie was wearing a dress that had an elastic em-
pire waistband, and as they all went to sit down, Marie's
elastic waistband broke and came flying out of the dress
and smacked the wife of the deceased right in the face.

GARY: Oh, boy.

YVONNE: Well, they just froze for a second, and then when
the widow burst out laughing, they followed. Chris said it
was such a tense moment and then when that happened,
it really lightened everything up. That's the point. To be
able to have a laugh or two even in the difficult times, es-

pecially in the difficult times, that helps us to cope with life. So, thank you, Chris for sharing your story. And, by the way, I welcome any and all stories—you can go to the website and email me with anything and you may hear it right here on WSEN.

Never Prejudge

GARY: How about a road story this morning?

YVONNE: On a recent flight to Milwaukee, a young girl sat in the seat next to me. She looked like any other teen, dressed in blue jeans and layered T-shirts, had the long hair, the backpack, the iPod. I totally prejudged her to be a spoiled teen who has everything and appreciates nothing.

We started to talk and she said she was seventeen and was going to visit a few colleges out west. Again, I thought, man! I'll bet she has no idea how lucky she is. To be able to get on a plane and go to college, you know. I never had that opportunity.

GARY: Yes. Right. A lot of us haven't.

YVONNE: I asked her what she hoped to do with her life, and I expected some pie-in-the-sky answer or the usual, "I don't know." But, boy, was I surprised! She said she was looking at several colleges but that eventually she wanted to work in Missions and help less fortunate people to have better lives. What a remarkable, kindhearted, young woman she was. So, this week I just wanted to share that story with your listeners to say that we really shouldn't prejudge simply by the way a person is dressed or their age, because you never really know—you could be sitting next to an amazing individual just like I was on that plane. This young girl was really an absolute inspiration to me. And she gave me a reason to be really proud of our young people.

GARY: You know, my grandfather was a union carpenter, but when he would go to work, he would wear a suit and tie and a hat. He worked at the State Tower Building, and the women told me they thought for years that my grandfather was a doctor or lawyer because he used to dress up to go to work. But then he would go down to his shop and put on his coveralls. When he finished work, he took the coveralls off and he put his suit back on. So, you're right. They prejudged him the other way. They thought this guy must be a doctor or lawyer just by the way he was dressed.

YVONNE: Isn't that great! Well, we can think about that this week and not be so eager to judge people by the way they look.

Technologically Challenged

GARY: I was talking to you the other day and you said you were going to get a new computer. Did you get one?

YVONNE: I got a MacBook and I'm so excited. I haven't even taken it out of the box yet, because I don't know how to turn the thing on. I'm very technology-challenged. I'm going to the Mac Store for lessons, so I should be up to speed soon. I come from a low-tech family, Gary. Mostly women in our family and we just don't know how to work anything. In fact, when we had the VCRs and the power went out, I used to put black electric tape over it so I didn't have to see that blinking light. The kids would come home and reset it for me. Last week, I was riding in the car with my mother and sisters. We were running late for a funeral. Everyone was getting all upset about being late and worried that our cousins would think we weren't coming. Everyone was all talking at once and driving me nuts. I calmly took out my cell phone and dialed 411 and asked for the funeral home's number. Then called the funeral home and asked that they tell our cousins we were in a traffic jam, but we were on our way. I got off the phone and my sister said, "What did you just do?" I said, "I called the funeral home." She said, "You know the number by heart?" I said, "No honey, I called 411." She said, "Wow, you got a good phone. My phone doesn't have 411." I said, "Do you have a four on your phone?" She said "Yes." "Do you have a one?" "Of course." "Well, then, you have 411!" "Ohhhhhh, I see."

GARY: Come on!

YVONNE: I'm not lying, Gary, that's how it happened. But that's not all. I think my mother is the only person on the planet who doesn't have call waiting. I hate calling over there and getting a busy signal. Where do you ever get a busy signal anymore?

GARY: Nowhere anymore.

YVONNE: Call my mother's house. You'll get a busy signal. I hate calling over there and getting a busy signal because you worry, you know. Did she fall down? Is something wrong?

GARY: Yep.

YVONNE: I'm telling you, the other day, for one hour that phone was busy. I got in the car and went over and I walked in. I said, "Ma, I've been calling you for an hour! You gotta get call waiting." She says, "I got call wait...you call, I'm talking, you wait, call wait!"

The Friendly South

GARY: You just got back from down South, right?

YVONNE: I was working in Tennessee. I actually was staying with a friend down there for a few days. We went to go run some errands and backed out of the garage and down the street. Every car that passed us waved and some honked the horn. My friend just waved back, and I said, "Boy, your neighbors are really friendly." She said, "Yes, they are just great." Then a third car passed and he laid on the horn and waved rather frantically and we both waved back and smiled. I said, "Every car has tooted and waved at you. Do you know these people real well?" She said, "Oh, no, honey. That's the Southern way. We're just really friendly." Finally, just as we were about to leave the neighborhood, a guy really laid on his horn and we honked back and passed him. He backed up his car and stopped, so she said, "Oh, that's my neighbor. He must have to tell me something. So she stopped the car and put it in reverse and just as she did her purse flew off the top of the car and slid down the windshield. Everything in it went flying onto the pavement. We just cracked up. Here she was so proud to think how friendly they were and they were trying to tell us we were idiots and left the purse on the top of the car. The lesson in this is things are not always what they seem. But, honey, we laughed a lot over that.

Easter Surprise

GARY: I'll tell you, the time is flying by. It's Easter already. How about some Easter traditions? You got anything special you do at Easter?

YVONNE: I do. I make a ricotta pie.

GARY: Nice.

YVONNE: I love it with the chocolate. You know, our family, we love to cook. We love to eat. My most memorable Easter was the year my mother made some extra-special Easter eggs. Every year, she paints the eggs for the kids, but this year she really took her time and made really beautiful eggs. She had flowers and bunnies and they were really masterpieces. They were like works of art. I remember when we got to the house, we saw the eggs and everyone was so impressed. We all commented on how she really spent so much time on these eggs, making each one special for each grandchild. And after dinner, we sat around the dining room table having our coffee and dessert. All the kids ran and got their special egg from grandma. Here they sit with their little salt shakers—twelve little kids sitting around the table. They each have their special egg.

GARY: Wow.

YVONNE: Well, I wish you could have seen the faces of these kids as each one cracked the shell of the egg to find...grandma had forgotten to boil the eggs.

GARY: Oh, no.

YVONNE: They're all crying. The egg drips down their little hands. We all just burst into laughter and Mom said, "Oh, dear, I must have forgot to boil the eggs." We just died laughing, so that is something we think about every Easter.

Massage Table Fall-Out

GARY: Alright, Yvonne, I know that you were on the road for a few days last week. Do you have any road stories? You always have a good road story for us.

YVONNE: I went to Boston last week and I was working with a very high-powered group of people and I was gone for several days. I'm a pretty relaxed, down-to-earth person when I am at home, but when I'm out there working out of town at these big conventions, I'm dealing with all these highly sophisticated, well...I call them big shots. So, I try hard not to say something stupid and act like an idiot. But no matter how hard I try to be sophisticated and polished, my true self always emerges, you know? I can't help it. I've got to be me. So I'm out of town. I'm exhausted. This woman that I'd been working with suggested that we go get massages after the conference. I thought, Gee, a massage would feel really good right now. We go to this fancy spa and it's so relaxing with the fountains, the soft music, and the scented candles. It's beautiful. She introduces me to the masseuse and we go into our separate rooms. I lay down on the table, and this gal is doing such a great job—so good that I fell asleep.

GARY: Yeah, okay, that was a good job.

YVONNE: Honestly, I was completely relaxed.

GARY: You were a piece of spaghetti, huh?

YVONNE: I was, I was. So much so that she had to actually nudge me and wake me to tell me to turn over. That's how good this girl was. She lifts the sheets so that I can roll over, but I'm so disoriented because I just woke up and I can't see because it's dark, that I roll away from her, instead of towards her and I fall off the table. Here I am, this woman is a nervous wreck. She drops the sheet and grabs one of my feet and one of my arms to keep me from hitting the floor. She was quick. Here I am hanging off the table, naked as a jaybird. I mean, how do you recover from that kind of humiliation? All I could do is laugh. So she says, "Are you alright?" I say, "Oh, honey, this happens to me all the time. My life is a never-ending sitcom. Let's just get back on the table and finish this up." So we get back in the car to head back to the hotel and the woman that I was working with, well, she had to have heard all the commotion. You know, when an elephant falls. Well, she asks me, "What was all that racket in there?" And I said, "Oh, that. That was my self-esteem falling off the table." Boy, we got a good laugh over that.

So the message for today is be yourself, don't try to be anything you're not, because truthfully, your true self always shines through, and mine certainly did that day.

Slip on the Stairs

Gary: Okay, Yvonne, you're always telling us a good story about your family. You always tell a story about your mother, great stories about your sisters that are so funny, your daughter, and your grandchildren. How about a family story this week?

Yvonne: I actually have a good one. There was a little bit of a disaster in our family this week, but it turned out to be great because of the kids in the family. You know, sometimes we take life so seriously because we have responsibilities, and demands, and deadlines. Life gets so serious, but I've always said that if we could just see things the way that kids do, we can get through anything. This week was a real reminder of that. I was visiting my daughter Aubry, and, as you know, she's got the three boys. I was coming down the stairs and I had just put my foot on the first step upstairs and somehow lost my footing.

Gary: Oh, boy!

Yvonne: I fell down a full flight of stairs. And I mean I hit every step, and I was screaming every time I hit. "Ow! Ow! Ow!" Screaming all the way down. I was thinking, Oh, boy, that's it, I'm breaking my hip and now they'll put me in a home. I hit every step with tears in my eyes, because it hurt. Well, I get to the bottom step, and my little two-year-old grandson Joe, who's at the top step, says, "Me go now, Nonni, my turn?" And I'm telling you, it just cracked us up. So I said, "Somebody throw that kid down the stairs. Make him happy, alright?" Of course, it wasn't fun to fall down the stairs, but when Joey made that comment, we just all laughed so hard, and it really helped because you really can't experience joy and pain at the same time. That little kid was able to erase my pain and I really appreciated that. It turned a bad situation into something that actually was kind of funny.

So my advice this week is sit at the kid's table and look at life from a different perspective.

Memorial Day

GARY: Okay, Yvonne, Memorial weekend coming up. Man, time is flying right by us.

YVONNE: It is, it really is. We are planning to go over to my daughter's and have a picnic. We've always had picnics with the family. So it's time. It's Memorial Day. You get out the grill, the lawn chairs, and start having some fun in the backyard. But really, this is a day for remembering those that have lost their lives to protect our country, and sometimes I think we are so into the picnic that we forget what the real reason is behind it. I happened to ask my mother one time what type of celebrations they had when she was a kid. My mother is eighty-four years old, so it's quite a while ago, but I was kind of surprised at her response, because I would think, Did they have picnics back then? What did they do?' She remembers a very special tradition that her town had. She grew up in a small town in Pennsylvania and her family and everyone else in this small town where she grew up would walk from the church to the cemetery carrying flowers to honor the veterans who had lost their lives in service to our country. Isn't that amazing?

GARY: Nice tradition, yes.

YVONNE: She said it was a very solemn walk. They walked really slowly and she said it was really a moving experience for her as a small child to take that walk to the cemetery and then to see all the flags that marked the graves of those who made the ultimate sacrifice. So, maybe this year, take a minute and talk to the seniors in your family and ask them to tell you about how they celebrated this holiday or really any other holiday in the past, and what this day really means to them. The memories add an interesting kind of flavor. When you talk about the past and you share your stories with the family, it's amazing. It's fun to see the grandchildren listening because this is so foreign to them, you know, anything the grandparents have to say. The children are so interested in what she had to say. Actually, the great-grandkids in our family. Older people have so much to tell us because they have lived an entire lifetime, but I think we have to let them know that we're interested to get them started. My mother would have never told that story if we didn't ask her about it, so once you get them started, you'll be surprised at what they have to say. So fire up the grill, and while the sausage is sizzling, ask your family to tell you a story about the way they have celebrated in the past and you may be surprised at what you learn.

Random Good Deed

GARY: Okay, Yvonne, here you are this week and you're bringing in a nice big batch of cookies. What did you think it was, my birthday or something today or what?

YVONNE: No, you know I just thought you might enjoy a treat and the staff here at the radio station would have a nice little dish of cookies during their break. It all started earlier this year when for Lent, instead of giving something up, I decided that I was going to do one random good deed, a random act of kindness, whatever you want to call it, each day. It was such a positive experience that I decided that I'm just going to continue this indefinitely and every day do something kind or something unexpected and nice for someone else. It's just such a wonderful feeling to do that because serving others actually makes us feel good about ourselves. We know it's the right thing to do, first of all. You think, Wow! I did the right thing. But it could be something as simple as opening a door for someone, or helping someone with a baby stroller that's at the mall. Have you ever seen these mothers with the strollers trying to get through the door? If you go over and hold that door open, they are just so grateful. Just the look on somebody's face, the gratitude, it's priceless. Letting someone go ahead of you in line.

Just recently I was in the grocery store and this little old lady—she broke my heart even just looking at her, because she looked like all my old relatives with the kerchief over her head—she's standing in front of me in line and she was a few dollars short and she had to put a package of chicken back. My heart just stopped and I'm like, Oh, dear Lord, this poor woman, she can't have her chicken. So I pulled a couple of dollars from my purse and I said, "Please allow me to bless you today," and I handed the clerk the money. The little old lady was so surprised, she just thanked me over and over and she left and I thought to myself, "Oh, I'm so grateful I had that opportunity to help this poor little old lady who wasn't going to get her chicken this week." The funny part is, I was out of the store and she gets into her brand new Lincoln! But the truth was, I got a good laugh out of it, so it kind of taught me that it doesn't really matter if a person needs your help or not. It's about giving. It's about being generous and kind and loving to other people no matter what. You can look for opportunities to serve others—it's everywhere—but the more you give to others, the more you serve others, the better your life will be. It really does come back to you tenfold.

My advice this week would be to do something kind and unexpected and nice for someone else.

GARY: Okay, and if you want to be nice the next time you come in, I'll have a big bowl of *pasta fagioli*.

YVONNE: Ooooh, okay.

Mail for Mom

GARY: Alright Yvonne, you know my mother's birthday is coming up this month and you're always really good at giving gifts. I need a little help now. I've run out of things to give my mom and you always come up with good stuff.

YVONNE: Well, I tell you. You know what I did for my mother's birthday in March? The thing we did for her was the best, best surprise I think we ever thought of, and it worked beautifully. She turned eighty-four and I thought what do you get an eighty-four year-old woman? She's got everything right? You want to try to declutter the house, not add more to it. I thought, This woman loves to open mail. I've never seen anybody more interested in mail than older people. They just love to open mail. It's like communication from the outside world and it's a big thing. I emailed all my friends and I said, "My mother's birthday is coming up; she loves to open the mail. If you feel it in your heart, send her a birthday card. Here's the address. I'm trying to get as many birthday cards sent as I can, sent to my mother." Gary, I can't tell you the people that sent cards. She got over a hundred birthday cards. It was amazing, and the joy that it brought her. It was like three weeks that she started to get the cards and it was so funny because she would get the cards and she didn't know who these people were. She would ask me and I would say, "Oh those are people from my church." Then she'd say, "Oh, how'd they remember it was my birthday? God bless them." In my head, I'm laughing, it was so funny. Then she'd say, "Oh, so and so must have told so and so it was my birthday." She'd make up all these things until finally she realized, Hey, I'm getting twenty cards a day, thirty cards a day, something is going on here. She came in one day and she said, "What did you do, threaten your friends?" We just laughed and laughed one afternoon. The thing is she really looked forward to it.

Every day my sister would take her to the post office to get her mail so she could see her cards. Donna told me, "Oh, you don't know. She rips those cards open. She can't even wait until we get home. She opens them in the car, she's so excited." Many people wrote beautiful notes and interesting things. It just warmed my heart to see her get so excited about the cards. One day she's opening the cards—she's got a stack of about twenty to twenty-five—and she says, "Oh, my goodness, the Post Office is going to be wondering what's going on." Between my sisters and myself and my mother we have been laughing for three solid weeks over that.

I told my hairdresser about it, and she says her sister did the same thing. When she turned fifty, her sister started sending her cards, so for three months before she turned fifty she got a card every day. Her sister works at a Hallmark Store, so she got really interesting cards like "Happy 90th Birthday," "Happy 100th Birthday." Then she got Chinese cards and cards in different languages. It was just hysterical and a prolonged way to have joy. You are laughing every day at the cards you get. Sending cards is an awesome thing. She said she got a big box of cards and she's having all of her clients sign the cards and she keeps them. Then when it's her sister's birthday, she's going to send hundreds of cards on one day.

GARY: Great idea, yeah.

YVONNE: Imagine what it feels like to get all those cards on your birthday! You know, do that with your mom. Just ask your friends to send cards. It's a wonderful gift. My mother really got so much joy out of that. She just loved it. She even put them all on the wall like you do Christmas cards. She had a hundred cards on her kitchen wall. It was hysterical. It was just one of the best things I think we've ever done.

Father's Day

GARY: Well, I'll tell you, Yvonne, this year is really flying by. Father's day already, this weekend coming up. I know a lot of folks have a lot of plans. How about you, anything special?

YVONNE: Actually, I'm going to go and be with my daughter and her husband and celebrate Father's Day there. We used to always go over to my dad's. You know, the whole family would go and spend the whole day there. We'd have a great big dinner and a celebration. Things are a little bit calmer than they used to be, but you know I was always proud to be my father's daughter. I've always had a great admiration for him and great respect and I think every father should have that as a goal for their children to look at them like that. Recently, I saw what I thought was the perfect description of what a father really is. I happened to catch my little two-year-old grandson Joey while he was walking down the driveway with his father.

His little hand was curled around his father's fingers and my son-in-law was talking to him. As they were going down the driveway, I really couldn't hear what Todd was saying, but I saw little Joseph looking up at his dad with complete trust and admiration. He had a big smile on his face and I heard him look up at his dad and say, "Wow, Daddy." It was so cute, and I thought, that's what a father is. He's someone that a little child can look up to with trust and admiration. Someone to really be amazed with, that's what a good father is. It reminded me of a song by Paul Peterson. I don't know if you remember, he used to be on the Donna Reed Show?

GARY: Sure, yeah.

YVONNE: He sang a song that was called "My Dad." At the end of that song, the lyrics say, "My dad, I love him so, and I only hope that someday, my own son will say, my dad, now there is a man." So if you have a child, keep in mind that he looks up to you and that whatever you say and whatever you do, it makes an impact. Be sure your example is a good one, and one that your child will remember with pride how he one day looked up at you, and said, "Wow, Daddy." Happy Father's Day.

Cemetery Laughter

GARY: Alright, Yvonne, you've always told me great stories about your mother. I feel like I know her and I love hearing stories about your mom. How about a story about your mom this week?

YVONNE: Well, you know, actually, something happened yesterday that just cracked the family up. We oftentimes will go up to the cemetery and fuss with the flowers and take care of the family that's up there. When we go, we like to go as a group. Of course, in my family, we don't do anything unless everybody goes. So my sisters, my nieces, and my mother, we're up there at the cemetery. We pull a few weeds and we plant a plant. Then we usually gather around and say a prayer before we leave. At that point, my sister Jackie—she's a little emotional—she always starts to well up with the tears. I try to keep it upbeat and positive. She says, "Vonnie, you say the prayer." We bow our heads and I say, "Dear Lord Jesus, we pray you have Daddy in your loving arms and that you forgive him for any sins and that he's with you now, without any pain, in your loving arms." Then my mother says, "Make room for me because I'm gonna be there soon." I'm trying to keep it light and it was kind of awkward when she said that. Right away Jackie starts crying. So I say, "Yes, Lord, make a nice comfy place for Mom and pour her a nice cup of tea." My mother says, "Never mind the tea, pour me a glass a scotch." We were like, "Mom you don't drink. What are you talking about?" We're all dying laughing. So she says, "I had enough tea. When I get to heaven I think I'm gonna need a good stiff drink, and I want scotch!" I mean, it took this scene from a little sad moment to something hysterical. Jackie called me three times last night laughing, "Can you believe mom said that about the scotch?" She just comes up with these things out of the blue, and totally out of character for her.

It just proves that no matter what the situation is, you can find something to laugh about that can really turn any situation around. Be laughing with your family this week and have some fun.

Fourth of July

Gary: Well, alright, Yvonne, here we are in just about the middle of summer here with the Fourth of July, another holiday weekend. Any special plans?

YVONNE: Well, you know, my sister Donnarae has a Fourth of July party pretty much every year. It's like no other Fourth of July party you will ever go to. Everybody has to come in costume. You have to be either George Washington, Betsy Ross, or one year I was the Statue of Liberty. I'm telling you, we go all out. I had a torch and the whole deal.

GARY: A Fourth of July theme party.

YVONNE: A Fourth of July theme party. Then we play charades or we play different kinds of games and she has gifts wrapped up in red, white, and blue. Most of the gifts are Fourth of July theme gifts as well. It's really kind of an interesting thing. If you win the games, you win different gifts. It's just a lot of fun. All the food is red, white, and blue. We have a cake that looks like the flag.

GARY: So, a serious theme party.

YVONNE: Oh, it's serious. We really do have a ball. If you don't wear a costume, then you have to get up and tell a story that maybe we might not know about. It has to do with some figure in history. This year I've got a good story about George and Barbara Bush. I don't know if you've ever heard this before, but it's supposedly a true story. They were traveling through Texas in the presidential motorcade and they stopped for gas. Have you ever heard this story?

GARY: No.

YVONNE: Okay, good. So the guy runs out of the gas station and can't wait to pump the gas for the presidential motorcade. He's all excited. Then, immediately, Barbara jumps out of the car, hugs this guy, and they begin to have this really nice chat. The president is in the car thinking, "Who the heck is this guy?" She gets back into the car and waves goodbye to the gas station attendant and off they go. As they drive away, George asks her, "Who was that guy?" She says, "That was my high school boyfriend. And I'll tell ya, I almost married him." Then the president says with a smirk, "Let me get this straight. You are married to the most powerful man in the world and you almost ended up marrying a gas station attendant?" And Barbara Bush looks at him and says, "Oh, George, don't be silly. If I would have married him, *he'd* be president."

So that just goes to show you, you never know what might end up happening. So have a good Fourth of July and maybe start a new tradition with your family and have a theme party and enjoy the day and learn a little bit about history.

Bastille Day

GARY: Alright, Yvonne, you tell me Bastille Day is coming up, another holiday. What the heck is Bastille Day, Yvonne?

YVONNE: Well, actually Bastille Day is a national holiday in France. It's the celebration of the storming of the Bastille, which was a French prison. It was actually the beginning of the French Revolution. It's a very big day in France, so they really celebrate extensively. When my children were little, we used to celebrate Bastille Day. I used to try to find different holidays from different countries and we would celebrate them. It was just kind of the way to teach my children about other countries. For instance, for Bastille Day, you could have French toast for breakfast, and French fries for dinner, or maybe go to a French restaurant, and just for fun, speak in a French accent. Like, "Oh, 'ullo, 'ow er you today?" It's just a fun thing to do with your kids. It's different, it costs you nothing, and they end up learning a little bit in the process. You can do it any time. You don't even have to wait until it's a holiday. We used to do silly things, like we would have theme dinners. Probably once a month I would do this with my kids. I'd say, "You pick a movie, and I'll cook a meal that has to do with that movie, and we'll dress up." One year, they picked "Gone With the Wind." That was my daughter's favorite movie. We dressed up. I actually took some old curtains and I was Scarlet and the kids picked characters from the movie and they went and found outfits, just something in the house. I cooked a big Southern meal complete with ham and pinto beans and homemade cornbread, and we spoke in a Southern accent. It was a ball. In fact, we videotaped that one. Sometimes, when the family gets together, we'll play those kinds of videos. Even my sisters shake their heads and say, "You are such a nut, Yvonne. The fact that your kids would even go along with you is crazy."

GARY: I think maybe some of our listeners would like to see that. Maybe you should get that up on YouTube.

YVONNE: Maybe I should. That's not a bad idea. But it's a great way to have fun with your kids. You know, we think that we have to spend a lot of money on our kids to make them happy, and I'm here to tell you that just is not true. You can have so much fun at home with your kids and they can learn something as well. It's a great way to bond with them and there is nothing like laughing your pants off with your kids. So have some fun this week with children.

GARY: Okay, and happy Bastille Day.

YVONNE: Thank you very much.

What's on Your Mind?

GARY: Yvonne, I know you have a story today about one of your local clients. Tell me about it.

YVONNE: I do, but first let me ask you. Have you ever gone somewhere, you're with people, and you think of something that would be really funny to say, but you stifle yourself, or you hold back because you're afraid that you might hurt somebody's feelings or something?

GARY: As a matter of fact, that happens a lot. Sometimes Krista will be looking at me and I'll try to hold something back and I'll just smirk and somebody will know and say, "Alright, what are you thinking?" Is that what you're talking about?

YVONNE: That's exactly what I'm talking about. Because in today's world, we're so concerned about being politically incorrect and oh, my goodness, you can't say this and you can't say that. I think a lot of the good and sponta- neous humor is stifled and we don't enjoy it. Really, the truth is, my father used to say the old sticks and stones will break your bones but names will never hurt you. We can't say that to our kids anymore because we are chang- ing the way we think about that sort of thing. My father always said, if you have a good self-image, if you know who you are, nobody can hurt you with words. I believe that's true. If you really think good of yourself, it doesn't matter what other people say.

Well, this story is about somebody that did not hold back. It's Christine, one of my clients, and she swears this is a true story. She said that during her church service her pastor was preaching on the topic of pain caused by evil. The pastor asked if they knew the devil was real, and this man stands up and says, "Of course, I know the devil is real. How quickly you forget that I've been married to your sister for over twenty years." The entire church burst out laughing. You see he saw an opportunity to have a little fun with the preacher and no doubt his wife would take it with a grain of salt because she knows who she is and has a good self-image. He just went for it. He saw something funny and he went for it. He was just poking fun, kidding. That's what was so funny about it. Christine said they really cracked up in the church and it made for quite a lively discussion on good and evil. The key is, if you really have a good self-image, then nothing anybody says in fun should be offending you.

Grace and Grey Poupon

GARY: Alright, Yvonne, here we are, and you know, I don't think I've heard a road story in a while. I think it's time for a road story this week.

YVONNE: I actually have two separate road stories. They are the best kinds. You know, when people come up to me at a conference and tell me a story, they're the best stories because they're spontaneous and fun. They are true stories and that's what really makes people laugh. This one comes from two nice Italian girls from Chicago. Mary Gaciono and Michelle Paciello. That's pretty Italian.

GARY: Yeah, I would say, yup.

YVONNE: Apparently, they were celebrating Michelle's fortieth birthday and they rented a limousine and really did the town. They're driving past cars and she said Michelle was such a ham, she rolled down the window and she's giving everybody the Queen Elizabeth wave, and just acting really silly and having a great time. They stop at a stoplight and she rolls down the window and there is a truck driver beside her, this big burly guy. She leans over and says with a British accent, "Excuse me sir, do you have any Grey Poupon?" The guy laughs and they drive on. Well, at the next stoplight the trucker toots the horn and hands her a jar of French's mustard that he happened to have in the cab. They just laughed and it was just one of those ongoing things where they went back and forth, laughing and having a good time.

She said that they also do all kind of fun things at work. They have a "bring a bag lunch day" where everybody brings their lunch in and they sit and watch funny DVDs or stand-up comics during lunch hour. It's a great way to kind of relieve the stress at work. Those people out in Chicago really know how to have fun.

I had another client tell me a funny funeral story. I love those. She said she's at her father's funeral. Her mother was just brokenhearted and so lost and she went slowly up to the casket, knelt down and made the sign of the cross and said a silent prayer. She steps away, faces the crowd, and then all of a sudden her sad face turns into the biggest smile and this little old lady bursts out laughing in front of all the mourners. Her daughter races up to her and says, "Mom, what's going on? Why are you laughing?" She says, "Oh, my goodness, I don't know what I'm doing. I think I just said Grace over your father." You know she's so used to saying the Grace over food. She didn't know what she was doing, so she said Grace. She said the whole room just cracked up when she said that. It broke the sadness of the moment.

You see, you can take even the saddest moment and turn it around with a good laugh. Once again, laughter is the best medicine.

21-Day Cleanse

GARY: Well, Yvonne, I've got to be real honest with you. You are looking really good. You've lost a lot of weight. What are you doing?

YVONNE: I'll tell you, it's the best thing I think I've ever done for myself is to lose this weight. I learned things about myself that I want to share with you and with the listeners because I know we all have troubles, we all have issues like this. Not just losing weight, but a lot of other things that we try to change in our life. I've always been a believer that we all have the power to change anything at all that we want about our life. It never worked for me when it came to dieting. I couldn't understand how come. I'm an intelligent person, I can change anything I want in my life, but when it comes to these measly ten pounds, I can't get rid of it. What's the problem? I think I figured it out. I think you have to attack losing weight as if it is a life-or-death situation, because that's what I did and it worked for me. I happened to go in for a physical and the doctor told me that my cholesterol was dangerously high, and she really scared me. She said, "Take a radical look at your life and tell me what you're doing that needs to be changed." I thought, Well, gee, you know, I eat pretty normal. I'm not an overeater. I have healthy food in my house. I really believed that I was doing everything I could. It just wasn't working. But she said to be radical. That kind of shook me up. When I took a truthful look, I had to admit, Hey, I eat a bowl of popcorn every single night because I think popcorn is the healthiest snack. I have a bowl the size of Texas and I cook it in oil, then I put in the salt, then I use the spray butter because that's better, but I spray every single kernel, so that's not so great. I ate that family-size bowl every single night. I started out the very next day after I had the conversation with the doctor and I decided to do what I'm calling my 21-day radical redirect. I knew that you could change any habit if you do something for 21 days. So for 21 days I ate fresh fruits, fresh vegetables, lentils, brown rice, and drank water. I had no coffee, no tea, no soda, and no red meat, anything with sugar. The good news is I lost 15 pounds in 21 days. I feel like I look great, and I feel great. My doctor was shocked when she saw me after I had the tests. My cholesterol was perfect. She said, "What are you doing? You're in perfect health. How did you do it?" She was shocked. She even asked me if I was taking medication. I said no. But I realized I had been poisoning myself with the food that I was eating without realizing it.

Every time I'd go to Aubry's, my daughter's, she's always got something good there to eat. I don't keep sweets at my house, but if I go to Aubry's I'll eat two or three cookies here, a piece of banana bread, you know, you don't think about it. Then, at our church, we have *more* food. If anyone is ever hungry, you need to go to The Vineyard because there is so much food there every time you go. So every time I go to church, I'm nibbling on chips, cookies—it's just a habit. And, of course, being Italian, whenever I visit with the family, even if I'm not hungry, I have to eat. So I changed the way I thought and I would say, "I'm sorry Mom, my doctor told me no sugar, no bad fats, no white bread, no white pasta." When you say "my doctor said," even an Italian mother will back off.

Just be radical about getting rid of any kind of bad habit. Not just the foods that you eat, but limiting myself to only fresh fruits and vegetables, and healthy choices, it really showed me all the stuff that I would have eaten if I weren't doing the 21-day challenge. It really makes you think. Honestly, you can change anything about yourself if you change the way you think. For me, it was just by saying that it was a life-or-death situation. It proves that you really can change anything, but you have to be radical. If you're the kind of person that never seems to get anything done, take your TV and give it away, that's pretty radical. If you're always getting into trouble, stop hanging around with bad people. You just have to say No, I'm done with this. If you can't seem to lose weight like I couldn't, stop eating crap. That's what I said, get all the junk out of your life.

You are always just one choice away from changing your life for the better. Philosopher William James said, "To change your life, start immediately, do it flamboyantly, with no exceptions, and no excuses." And I'll add: Be radical. It worked for me.

I'm Bored

GARY: Alright, Yvonne, I know you've talked about it before. You've got three grandsons, right?

YVONNE: Yes, three grandsons.

GARY: Yeah, they've got to keep you busy, huh?

YVONNE: They do, and especially during the summer. I just spend so much time with them because I work less in the summer than I do any other time of the year. I'm right there with the kids. We have a good time, but have you ever had a kid say to you, "I'm bored"?

GARY: Oh, all the time. I remember those days when my kids were growing up.

YVONNE: Nothing gets under my skin more than a kid that says "I'm bored." Because I'm thinking to myself that there is so much to do. You know, you're surrounded by games, computers, and every toy in the store. Kids today, they have everything, how could you possibly be bored? Last week I created a new game with my grandson that I would like to share with the listeners in case they have kids sitting around the house saying they're bored. It's called "What Are You So Happy About?" You can also use this game when your kids say, "Nothing ever works out for me," "Nobody likes me," "Johnny's picking on me." Any kind of complaint, you know, whenever a kid is whining or complaining.

GARY: This will come in handy.

YVONNE: Absolutely. Any kind of negative statement can be turned around with this game, and here's what you do. When you say to a kid, "What are you so happy about?," it kind of helps the kid focus on what's right in their world. What's going right? You actually can do this with adults, too. You take turns with your kids and you ask, "What are you so happy about?" For instance, I'm so happy I don't have to work tomorrow. Then my grandson will say, "Well I'm so happy that my homework is done." So you keep on stating back and forth what you are happy about until the kid starts to realize that, hey, life's really not so bad. You want to try this with me now, spontaneously?

GARY: Sure, go ahead.

YVONNE: I'll start and then you take a turn. Say what you're so happy about. I'm so happy that my sister is going to come and visit me this afternoon.

GARY: Alright. Well, I'm so happy to be here at work today, with you.

YVONNE: Well, thank you. And I'm so happy that I'm almost done and I'm going to be able to go home and spend some time out in the sunshine.

GARY: Well, I'm almost with you there, too.

YVONNE: You know it's just being grateful, basically, is what it is. You are teaching your children or whoever you're playing the game with that no matter what your troubles, there are still plenty of things to be grateful for. Cookies, a beautiful day, a great family, a nice house to live in, the dog, maybe your little brother is sleeping so you have more time with your mom. It's also a great little way to find out what your kids are thinking is good, because sometimes you'll be surprised at what they are grateful for or what makes them happy.

GARY: You know, I wish we had this game when I was a kid, because you know what my father used to say when I said I was bored? My father used to say, "Go grab a bag inside and I got some weeding you can do, if you're bored." My dad used to put us to work if we were bored. "I'll find something for you to do. Come here, cut the grass."

YVONNE: You know, I'll have to agree with you. That's exactly what my father and mother used to say. You're bored, get over here and clean the garage. You can either put your kids to work this week or you can play the "What Are You So Happy About" game and see if that turns their attitude around in a jiffy.

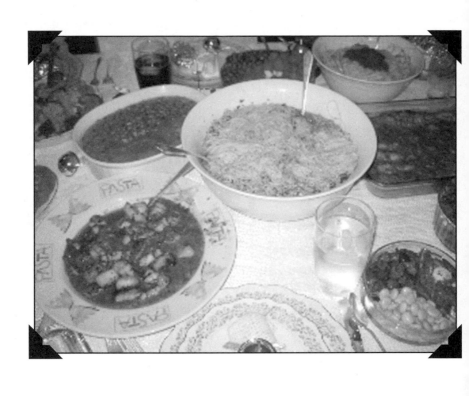

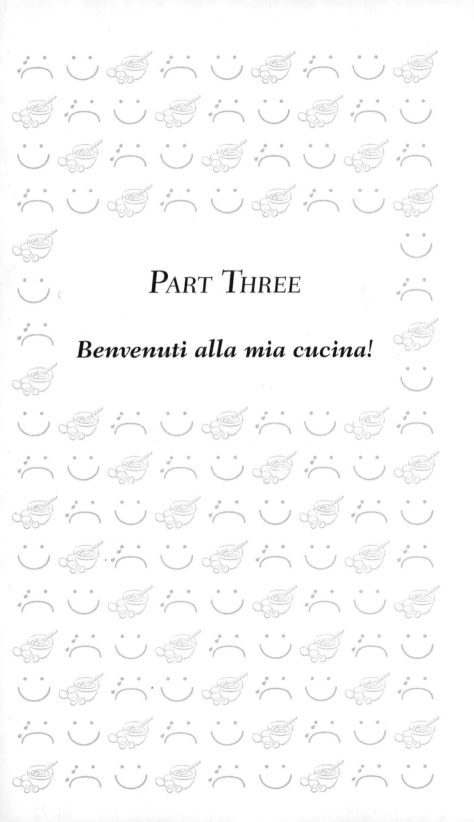

PART THREE

Benvenuti alla mia cucina!

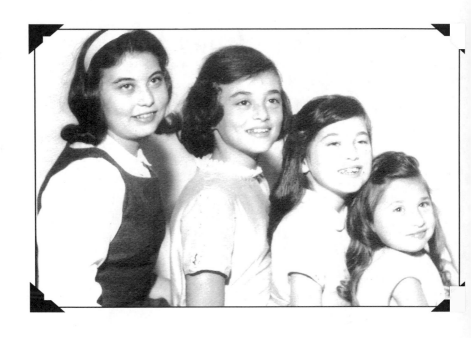

Donnarae, Yvonne, Jacqueline, and Anna Marie

Our family is known for our ability to cook, bake and entertain. We are Italian Americans and making a meal is not just something we do to keep ourselves healthy, it is part of our heritage to cook with passion. It is a creation. My father always referred to his food as 'beautiful; a beautiful piece of meat, a beautiful broth, a beautiful onion. It was all beautiful. I think it's because our grandmothers and great grandmothers really took pride in what they whipped up in the kitchen and they handed that pride down to, not only their daughters and grand daughters, but their sons and grandsons as well. These recipes *came over on the boat!* If you're a Conte, you can make a meal out of nothing! A little pasta, a few tomatoes and just about anything else will make a great meal!

My Grandparents had Conte's restaurant on Columbia Street in Utica, New York, and my Uncle Carl owned the North Genesee Club Diner in North Utica and in the '50s Elvis Presley and his entourage had breakfast there. He also ran the Diplomat Restaurant in Utica. My cousin Marilyn is a fixture up in Ogdensburg. Her restaurant, The Donut King, has been feeding the masses in the North Country for decades. The fact that my cooking roots simmered from Utica kitchens is a big deal. Everyone knows there is no better place on earth to get a good meal and a yummy pastry than Utica New York.

I can't explain the reason behind it except that many, many good recipes were created in Utica restaurants and everything just tastes better there. Maybe it's the water.

Please do not worry about calories, points or fat grams! Three thousand years ago the great Solomon said so! Look it up. "So go ahead. Eat your food and drink your wine with a happy heart, for God approves of this!" (Ecclesiastes 9:7). Just enjoy. If you live a joy-filled life and laugh a lot with family and friends, you wont gain weight. It's been proven that every time you laugh, you burn calories and exercise sixteen major organs in your body. *Mangia!*

Antipasto/Appetizers

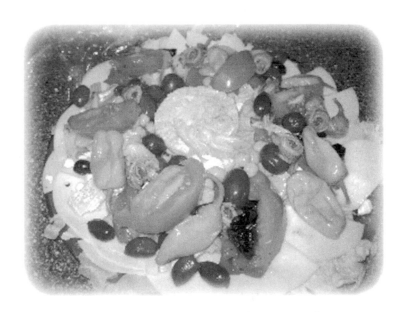

Funghi Imbolite alla Florentina
(Yvonne's Stuffed Mushrooms)

This is great as an appetizer or as a side dish to any good Italian meal.

1 pound fresh mushrooms
¼ cup onions, chopped fine
¼ cup seasoned Italian bread crumbs
8–9 ounces frozen spinach, thawed out
    and chopped
Olive oil
Salt and pepper

Preheat the oven to 350°F. Pull the stems from the mushrooms, chop them, and set aside. Be careful to keep the caps looking nice. Scoop out the meat of the mushroom and put with the stems. (I use a grapefruit spoon with a serrated edge.) Brush the caps with olive oil and set in a baking pan.

Heat about 3 tablespoons of olive oil in a pan and add the onions and mushrooms stems, and sauté. Stir in the bread crumbs, spinach, salt, and pepper, and spoon into the caps. Bake about 15 minutes.

Peperoni con Capperi

Sounds fancy, but it just means red peppers and capers. Simple, simple, simple.

7-ounce jar roasted red peppers
1 tablespoon capers

Lay your peppers nicely on a platter and sprinkle with the capers. It's just that easy, and it's a really pretty, colorful dish. Serve with some nice crusty bread.

Italian Potato Salad

My longtime friend and hairdresser, Cathy Zoccolillio-DeBello, gave me this recipe.

Little red potatoes, cooked and cooled
String beans, cooked and cooled
Olive oil
Garlic to taste

Sauté the garlic in olive oil and let cool. Pour over the potatoes and string beans and mix thoroughly. Refrigerate and serve cold.

Lupini

We eat these like candy. It's a nice little snack.

2 garlic cloves, chopped
1 jar lupini beans
Parsley
Olive oil
Red wine or balsamic vinegar

Combine all ingredients. Chill well before serving.

Spiedini di Verdure (Artichoke Kebabs)

1 jar marinated artichoke hearts
1 jar marinated mushroom caps
1 jar sweet fried red peppers
Long toothpicks

Drain and save the liquid from the jars. Cut the peppers into strips. Wrap a pepper strip around each artichoke piece and hold it with a toothpick. Stick a mushroom cap at the end of the toothpick. It's pretty, it's easy, and it's delish! Once you have them nicely arranged on a platter, drizzle the juices over the top.

Ceci in Insalata

I told my friend Barbara I'd like to make her some Ceci in Insalata. *She said, "Ceci Insalata? That sounds like a dance to me." Don't get nervous. It's just garbanzo beans, or, as some call them, chickpeas. We always called them ceci beans.*

⅓ cup olive oil
2 tablespoons fresh lemon juice
Oregano leaves, crushed
Salt and pepper
1 clove garlic, crushed
1 can ceci beans, drained
1½ cups ripe tomatoes, diced
¼ cup green pepper, chopped

Combine all ingredients in a bowl and serve chilled. This is really a beautiful dish.

Soup/Pasta

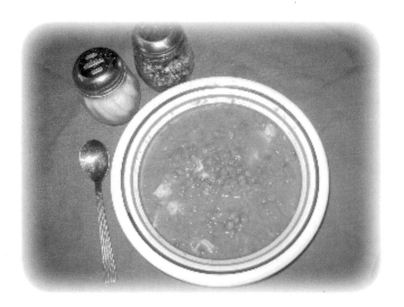

Zuppa di Pollo
(Nonni Vonnie's Chicken Soup)

I make chicken soup any time I feel a cold coming on.
I'm better in no time. Kale is great in soup. It's so good
for you, and gives it a nice full flavor. I cheat and use
a few cans of chicken broth—hey, at least I'm honest!

1 chicken, washed and cut up
3–4 carrots, peeled and sliced
3–4 stalks of celery, chopped
1 large onion, chopped
1 large tomato, chopped
7–8 leaves of kale or spinach, torn
Salt and pepper
Chicken broth

Cook the chicken in the broth until the meat falls off the
bone. Strain it and discard the bones and skin. Add the
vegetables and cook until soft. Add salt and pepper to
taste. You can add small pasta or rice to this, too.

Zuppa di Lenticchi
(Lentil Soup)

1 carrot, peeled and chopped
1 medium onion, chopped
2 stalks celery, chopped
2 cloves garlic, crushed
1 large tomato, chopped
Dried lentils
Beef or vegetable broth
Olive oil

Cook lentils in water for about an hour. Heat the oil in
a frying pan and sauté the carrots, onions, garlic, and

celery until the onion is tender. Add the tomato and cook a little more.

Pour all into a pot with lentils and cook until the lentils are soft. Serve with cheese and some good bread.

Cousin Nancy's Italian Wedding Soup

MEATBALLS

> 1 small onion, grated
> ⅓ cup chopped parsley (I use dried)
> 1 large egg
> 1 teaspoon minced garlic (I use jarred)
> 1 teaspoon salt
> 1 slice fresh white bread, crust trimmed off,
>   torn into small pieces
>   (Wonder Bread works best)
> ½ cup grated Parmesan cheese
> 8 ounces ground beef
> 8 ounces ground pork
> Freshly ground black pepper

SOUP

> 3 boxes chicken broth
> 1 pound curly endive, coarsely chopped
> 1 package pastini pasta

Mix all meatball ingredients except the meat in a bowl until well incorporated. Add the meat and roll into small balls.

Bring the broth to a boil and add the meatballs and endive. Continue cooking until meatballs are cooked through and the endive is tender.

Cook the pastini according to package directions and add to the soup.

Carla's Easy Sauce

I've been making sauce now for over 40 years. Carla gave me her recipe a while ago, and now I make it just like this every time. It's just so perfect.

> Pork ribs or spare ribs
> Garlic, chopped
> Fresh plum tomatoes or canned tomatoes
> 2 cans sauce to one can tomato paste
> Fresh basil
> Salt

Fry the meats with the garlic and add the tomato sauce and paste. (My Aunt Frances used to squeeze the tomatoes with her hands; I use the back of a wooden spoon.) Add the basil. Make up some meatballs and fry on top of the stove. Add to the sauce. Don't use too much oil—there shouldn't be an oil slick on top of the sauce. Simmer for a few hours. You may add 2 links of sweet Italian sausage, if you want, or chicken; it really doesn't matter. I never cover my sauce while it's cooking.

Frank Conte's Quick Clam Sauce

My father loved to cook. He loved to eat even more, and did both with gusto. Daddy always said the secret to good clam sauce is in the anchovies. He gave me this recipe on May 30, 1985.

> 1 can Progresso white clam sauce
> 1 can chopped clams
> 3 or 4 anchovies, mashed
> 1 clove garlic, minced
> Olive oil
> Fresh parsley, chopped

Heat olive oil and add garlic, stirring until softened. Do not brown! Add the anchovies, clam sauce, and chopped clams. Add lots of parsley and bring to a boil. Lower heat and simmer slowly, about 10 minutes. Pour over buttered linguini.

Aglio e Olio

I love this dish. It's the easiest pasta dish on the planet to make and one of my all-time favorites. My father taught me how to make this. I thought it must be so complicated because it was so darned good. I cracked up when I discovered how easy it was to make.

1 pound thin pasta
½ cup olive oil
5–6 cloves garlic, mashed
1–2 tablespoons red pepper, crushed

Cook the pasta al dente. Heat olive oil and sauté garlic and red pepper until garlic is just lightly browned. I add anchovies at this point, but that's just me. Remove from heat. Drain pasta but save a little water in case you need it. Toss together the pasta and sauce. You can add a tiny bit of pasta water if it seems too dry.

Peas and Macaroni

Any pasta
Fresh peas
Marinara sauce

This is another easy one. You make a marinara sauce and add some fresh peas and pasta. Bada-bing! You've got dinner. (You can use frozen peas if you want to.)

Gnocchi

I don't know the English word for this. It's just small, chewy pasta, but it is so amazingly good. You have to try it. I made these once for my dad and he cried he was so happy, and so proud of me.

4–5 pounds potatoes, washed and peeled
5–6 cups flour
Salt

Boil the potatoes and rice them completely. Little by little, add flour to the potatoes and knead until smooth and manageable.

Roll the dough into long ropes about ¾ of an inch thick. Cut the rope into 1-inch pieces. Take the prongs of a dinner fork and press down lightly on each piece to make it curl around. (I use my pointer finger.) It should look like a little shell when you are done. Toss them in boiling salted water for 10–12 minutes. Drain. Serve with your favorite tomato sauce and cheese.

Quick Fettuccine all' Alfredo

3 tablespoons butter
1 cup heavy cream
1½ cup Parmesan cheese
Salt and pepper
Pinch nutmeg
Parsley

Heat up butter and ¾ cup of cream until the butter is melted and it comes to a boil. Lower the heat and simmer a minute or two. Cook the pasta. Pour the hot pasta into the sauce and mix well. Add the remaining cream and one cup cheese, nutmeg, salt, and pepper. Top it off with more cheese and serve with red pepper and crusty bread. You can add bits of ham and peas to this, too, and it makes it really pretty. Garnish with parsley.

Pasta with Anchovies

The great thing about Italian cooking is that you can whip up a great meal in about ten minutes. All you need is some pasta, some olive oil, and almost any other ingredient.

½ cup olive oil
3 cloves garlic, minced
1 can anchovies, mashed, or anchovy paste
1 pound pasta (I like angel hair with this dish)
3 tablespoons seasoned Italian bread crumbs

Heat olive oil in a pan and add garlic and red pepper until garlic is lightly brown (not burned). Add anchovies or anchovy paste and bread crumbs. Mix well and heat through. Add cooked and drained pasta. Mix thoroughly and serve with grated cheese.

Vonnie's Good Italian Meatballs

Barbara says my meatballs are so good they'll cross your eyes. I've been making meatballs for my family for almost forty years. I love the smell they leave in the house. I have no idea who gave me this recipe but I am eternally grateful, because they really are the best meatballs in the world.

½ pound ground pork
½ pound ground veal
½ pound ground beef

2 slices *good* Italian bread
Milk
3 eggs
½ cup *good* fresh-grated Parmesan/Romano
    cheese
Handful parsley, chopped
Salt and pepper
½ cup onion, chopped

Tear the bread in tiny pieces and put in a bowl with the milk. Let it sit a while, then drain off the milk. Combine everything but the meats. Then mix in the meats with your hands until well blended. (By the way, don't buy that meatloaf mix they sell in the grocery store. Look at it. It's only 10% pork and 5% veal. It needs to be equal amounts of each meat.) Wet your hands and form the meat mixture into balls, adding more egg if necessary to hold the mixture together.

You can sauté the meatballs in olive oil on top of the stove, or you can bake them in the oven but this is how I do it: Roll the meatballs in seasoned bread crumbs and sauté in olive oil. OMG! They really are amazing. Nice and crispy on the outside and moist and delish on the inside. They freeze well, too.

Meatless Meatballs

Again, my friend Cathy gave me this recipe. At first I thought, How the heck do you make meatballs without the meat? You just use all the ingredients you usually use but leave out the meat and fry them in olive oil. I make small balls, skewer them with toothpicks, and serve with a marinara sauce for a tasty appetizer. Cathy makes them regular size and serves with any pasta dish. They are sort of the Italian version of Southern hush puppies.

Marinara del Estate
(Vonnie's Vegetable Marinara)

SAUCE

½ cup onion, chopped
2 cloves garlic, mashed
2 pounds fresh ripe plum tomatoes
    (or if no one is looking—canned tomatoes)
Salt and pepper
8 fresh basil leaves, torn
Splash of red wine

OTHER GOODIES

2 cups broccoli
2 cups zucchini
1 can chickpeas, drained
7-ounce jar roasted red peppers, diced
6-ounce jar marinated mushrooms
Handful fresh parsley

Heat some olive oil and sauté the onions and garlic until golden. Don't let them burn. Add tomatoes, salt, and pepper. Simmer until the sauce is thick. Add basil and wine and simmer another 5–10 minutes. This sauce is a little bland at this point, but wait until you add the rest….Mmmmm. At this point, this is actually a simple Marinara sauce.

In a very large frying pan put a little olive oil and cook the broccoli and zucchini briefly. They should still be crisp. Add chickpeas, peppers, mushrooms, and parsley. Add the marinara sauce. Serve over pasta with lots of Parmesan or Romano cheese.

Cicoria Fina Agliata
(Dandelion with Garlic)

My Great Uncle Carl used to pick us dandelions all the time. My father said he grew up on this.

2 pounds freshly picked dandelions,
    cleaned and cut
2–3 cloves garlic, mashed
Salt and pepper
Olive oil

Heat oil and garlic, add greens, salt, and pepper. Cook about 10–12 minutes and serve.

Primo Piatto/Main Course

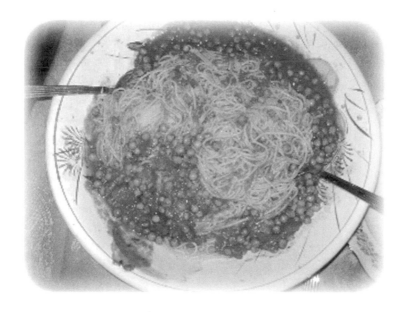

Chicken, Potato, and Carrots in the Oven

This was a staple in our family. If unexpected company came, my mother could whip this up in two minutes, and by time we hugged and kissed and set the table, dinner was ready.

Chicken parts—breast, legs, wings, whatever
Potato, cut in quarters with skins on
Carrots, cut in about 2-inch pieces
Onion, cut in chunks
Salt and pepper
Garlic salt
Parsley
Olive oil

Basically, you cut it all up, lay it in a baking pan, season it, and bake it. Done! My mother had a great little carrot cutter that made pretty jagged edges. I have one, too. I made carrot puzzles with it for my kids when they were little. You can cut your veggies any way you want. Sprinkle them with olive oil, salt, and pepper, garlic salt, and parsley and bake 45 minutes at 350°F.

Pollo Piccante
(Chicken Piccante)

I love this for company, because it looks so special and fancy. Everyone loves it. By the way, I always use Progresso brand, but you can use what you are used to.

6–8 boneless, skinless chicken breasts
¼ cup Italian bread crumbs
Rosemary
Oregano
Red pepper, crushed

Salt
Olive oil
1 cup dry white wine
3 cups mushrooms, sliced
2 cloves garlic, crushed
7-ounce jar roasted red peppers
2 teaspoons capers (more or less)
Handful fresh parsley, chopped

I pound my chicken flat—it just looks and cooks better, I think. Coat the chicken with bread crumbs and pan-fry in good Italian olive oil. Sauté until nicely browned on both sides. Sprinkle with seasonings. Pour the wine over the chicken and cook about 25–30 minutes. Just before the chicken is done, sauté the mushrooms and garlic in olive oil in a clean pan Add peppers and capers. Put the chicken on a platter and spoon the mushroom mixture over it. This is so beautiful, you'll want to take a picture. I serve this with the Vegetable Marinara Sauce and Pasta.

Utica Chicken Riggies

My cousin Carla Jonquil taught me how to make this dish. Carla and my cousin Nancy Pimpinella are some of the best cooks in the family. Carla's dad, my Uncle Carl Conte, and Nancy's father's brother Salvatore Gerace owned the Diplomat Restaurant in Utica for years. Any time I need to know how to make anything, I call either Carla or Nancy. Chicken Riggies is a great dish to make for company, because you can make most of it the day before and your kitchen isn't all hot and messy when the company comes. This is so good that Utica has a festival called Riggiefest to celebrate the unique dish. Each year, riggie aficionados crowd the festival to sample and vote for the area's best.

5 skinless, boneless chicken breasts
Garlic powder
Olive oil
2 medium onions, chopped
5 cloves garlic, minced
2 red bell peppers, cut into medium-size pieces
2 green peppers, cut into medium-size pieces
2 pounds mushrooms, sliced
16-ounce jar pepperoncini, cut up
    (reserve the juice)
Small can tomato paste
1 pound mini rigatoni
2 cups light cream
¼ cup of *good* Romano cheese

Preheat oven to 400°F. Sprinkle the chicken breasts with garlic powder and bake for 35–45 minutes. Cool and cut into bite-size pieces. Set aside.

Sauté the veggies in olive oil until just tender. Add tomato paste, reserved juice from the peppers, chicken, and Romano cheese. Mix well and refrigerate overnight.

Cook the rigatoni, drain, and add to the veggie-chicken mixture. Mix well. Add cream and heat thoroughly. Top with more cheese.

Scharole e Fagioli
(Escarole and Beans)

1 large head escarole, cleaned and chopped
Olive oil
2 cloves garlic, chopped
2 cups chicken broth
1 can cannellini beans

Sauté garlic in olive oil for about a minute. Add escarole, chicken broth, and beans. Simmer till the escarole is cooked and you've got what we always called *scharole*. You can add chicken to this if you want to.

Scharole e Aioli
(Escarole and Garlic)

1 head escarole, cleaned and chopped
3 cloves garlic, thinly sliced
Red pepper
Olive oil
Salt and pepper

In a soup pot, sauté the garlic and red pepper in olive oil until garlic is golden. Add the escarole, salt, and pepper. Stir. Cover and cook about 15 minutes.

Pasta e Fagioli
(Pasta and Beans)

We used to eat this on Friday without the meat when I was little.

1–2 pounds hot Italian sausage (optional)
2 carrots, chopped
2 celery stalks, chopped
1 onion, chopped
4 cloves garlic, chopped
1 bay leaf
Salt and pepper
Chicken broth or water
2 teaspoons tomato paste
Kidney beans or white beans
Parmesan/Romano cheese
Ditalini pasta

Brown sausage, and add veggies and bay leaf. Pour in broth (it makes it richer than water) and beans. Add pasta. As soon as the pasta is al dente, it's ready. Serve with lots of cheese and some red pepper. You can add rosemary to this or thyme if you like that.

Utica Greens

1 large head escarole, cleaned and
    chopped into large pieces
4 thin slices prosciutto, chopped
2 cloves garlic
2 long hot peppers, seeded and sliced
Olive oil
¼ cup Romano cheese
½ Italian bread crumbs
8–10 ounces chicken broth
Salt and pepper

Boil the escarole till it's wilted. Sauté garlic and prosciutto in olive oil a few minutes. Do not burn the garlic. Add the peppers and cook another minute. Add the escarole, salt, pepper, and chicken broth. Gradually add the bread crumbs and cheese on top. Toss lightly to blend. Put it in a casserole dish with some bread crumbs on top and run under the broiler for about 3–5 minutes. Serve hot.

Fiori di Zucca Fritti
(Fried Squash Flowers)

This was one of my favorite things to eat in the spring-time. Aunt Jenny taught me how to do this at camp.

2 handfuls flour
2 handfuls Parmesan cheese

Squash flowers, washed and torn
Pepper
Eggs
Milk

Whisk a few eggs and some milk together and add the flour, cheese, and pepper. Mix well. It should be like wallpaper paste. Dip the flowers in the batter and slip them individually into some hot, hot oil and fry, turning once, until both sides are golden brown. Drain on paper towels or brown paper bags and serve immediately, while still nice and crisp.

Sausage and Peppers

My little Southern friends just love this dish, but to us Conte's, this is nothing new. We've been eating this at every wedding, shower, graduation, confirmation, and holy communion party in the family. You can serve this on its own with some crusty Italian bread to soak up the delicious juices. Always use the best Italian sausage you can find and the freshest peppers. I always make this for a really large group, but I will try to cut it down to a normal family size for you.

2 rings Italian sausage, hot, sweet, or mixed,
    cut in 2-inch pieces
6–8 sweet green and red peppers, cut in strips
1 medium onion, sliced really thin
3 cloves garlic
Olive oil
Salt and pepper
Handful of fresh parsley

Brown sausage on both sides. Add the onions and cook until they are nearly translucent. Add the peppers and garlic and cook till the peppers are tender and the sausage is well done, about 20–30 minutes. Remove from heat. Add some salt, pepper, and parsley, and serve. Sometimes I just put it all together and bake it in the oven at 450°F. You can do that, too.

Great Aunt Jenny's Dinner

My Great Uncle Carl and Great Aunt Jenny Conte had a wonderful camp on Canadarago Lake in Otsego County. Truth be told, the camp actually belonged to cousins Frances and Sam Paone and was called the Jan-Ricky Camp after their children, but everyone in the family referred to the camp as Aunt Jenny and Uncle Carl's camp. I loved going there and seeing the family. On any given Sunday, they had at least twenty people around the table for dinner. And you really never knew what you were eating, because Uncle Carl and cousin Hank liked to hunt. We ate whatever they caught: woodchuck, rabbit, squirrel, deer—we never asked, we just ate it. Aunt Jenny and Frances's sauce could make anything taste great. This dish is one that I can taste just thinking about it. We just called it Aunt Jenny's Dinner. She used to can it and always gave us several jars to take home. You can put any veggie from the garden in this. It's sort of like a veggie stew. You can also add meat to it if you want.

    Green beans
    Onions
    Yellow squash
    Zucchini
    Garlic
    Fennel
    Celery leaves

Tomatoes
Parsley

Sauté the onions and garlic in olive oil. Add the fresh chopped tomatoes, parsley, basil, fennel, celery leaves, and simmer. Add some yellow squash or zucchini, a little salt and pepper, and Mmmmmm!

Aunt Jeanette's Pork Chops

I loved to go to my Aunt Jeanette's house. She was always so nice to me and had such a beautiful smile all the time. She was a great cook and passed that down to her children. My cousins were all a few years older than me and I liked being with the big kids. This is one of her specialties.

1 package Uncle Ben's long-grain wild rice
6 thick chops, with a pocket sliced in the side
(ask your butcher to do it for you)
Flour
Salt and pepper
Butter
Olive oil
1 small jar or can sliced mushrooms
¼ cup white wine

Preheat oven to 350°F. Prepare rice but cook it only 20 minutes. Stuff the chops with rice and skewer with toothpicks. Dust with flour, salt, and pepper. Pan fry about 5 minutes on each side in oil and butter. Arrange in a buttered casserole dish. Add to the frying pan any reserved liquid from the rice and mushrooms and top off with water to make one cup. Add the mushrooms and wine. Pour over the chops and bake about 1 hour.

Cousin Nancy's Baked String Beans

My Aunt Frances lived in Utica, where I once sold phone systems. I always stopped at Aunt Frances's house because I knew I would get a great meal and I would laugh a lot. She usually made me a great big salad made with garlic, fresh basil, olive oil, and red wine vinegar. It was so good I wanted to lick the bowl. She used to make me these string beans. Now her daughter—my cousin Nancy—makes them. She taught me how to make them but I have to say...Nancy's taste better than mine. You can do this with almost any vegetable.

Whole fresh string beans
Salt and pepper
Olive oil

Preheat the oven to 350°F. Clean your veggies, put them on a cookie sheet, sprinkle with salt, pepper, and olive oil and bake uncovered a few minutes. I like them a little burnt, but you do it the way you want. Sometimes I put a little garlic salt on them, too.

String Beans and Tomato

Fresh string beans, cut into bite-size pieces
Olive oil
2 cloves garlic, chopped
1 medium red onion, chopped
2 ripe tomatoes, diced
2 splashes red wine vinegar
Fresh basil,chopped and crushed
Red pepper, crushed
Salt and pepper

Cook beans for a few minutes (should be crisp). Set aside. Sauté onion and garlic until soft. Add tomatoes, vinegar, red pepper, salt, and pepper and stir. Cook 3–4 minutes. Add basil and beans. Cook another few minutes.

Daddy's Cheesy Potato

One of the best tips my dad gave me in the kitchen was to use up all your leftovers. He just added little bits of stuff to anything and it worked. Next time you're making mashed potatoes, look in the fridge and see what you have that can be thrown in for flavor.

8–10 potatoes
Handful Parmesan cheese
Scoop ricotta cheese
Chicken stock
Salt and Pepper

Cook potatoes. Leaving the skins on, mash them up. (My father always told us the best part of the potato is the skin.) Add a handful of Parmesan cheese and a scoop ricotta cheese, some chicken stock, salt, and pepper. Whip it up. These are really good with Aunt Jeanette's pork chops.

Cotolette di Vitella
(Veal/Chicken Cutlets)

1 pound veal or boneless, skinless chicken,
    pounded flat
2–3 eggs
Handful Pecorino cheese, grated
2 cups bread crumbs
Sweet fresh basil, chopped

Olive oil
Salt and pepper
Lemon

Mix the bread crumbs, cheese, basil, salt, and pepper. Roll the meat in the crumbs, then dip in the egg and then back into the crumbs. Brown the meat on both sides in hot oil. Lower your heat and cover them. Cook for about 20 minutes or until done. Drain any excess oil. Serve with lemon slices.

Dolce/Dessert

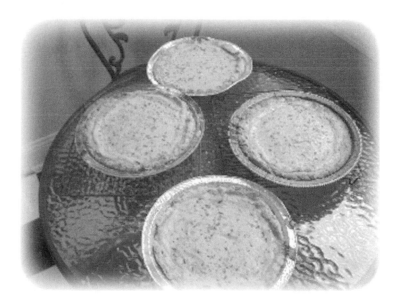

Jackie's New York Cheesecake

This is my sister Jackie's specialty. She makes them every time we get together for something special. Everyone knows Jackie by the delicious baked goods she cooks up in her kitchen, but this one beats them all! I've been asking her for this recipe for almost thirty years. She always says, "Yes, sure, okay, I'll get it for you." But then somehow she "forgets" to give it to me. I didn't realize all I had to do was write a cookbook and she would hand over the goods, but that's just what happened. If I knew that, I would have written this book years ago!

    2 recipes graham cracker crust
    3 8-ounce packages cream cheese
    5 eggs
    1¾ cups sugar
    2 tablespoons vanilla
    1 quart sour cream

Preheat oven to 375°F. Follow the recipe on a box of Honey Maid Graham Cracker Crumbs to make two recipes. Cream the cheese well, then add the sugar. Whip it up nice and creamy. Keep the beaters going and add eggs one at a time. Mix in some sour cream and add vanilla a little at a time. Pour into a 9 × 3 springform pan and bake for 40 minutes.

Shut off the oven and keep the door closed, letting the cake stand in the oven for one hour. Chill when cooled. Refrigerate one day before cutting. You can put any kind of fruit on this once it's cold or serve plain. It's soooooo goood!

Cousin June's Italian Drop Cookies

June gave this to Nancy and Nancy gave it to me. I remember June's cookies and, Mama mia! They are wonderful. Only an Italian would make this many cookies at one time, but June was Italian only "by association."

4 sticks butter
2 cups sugar
12 eggs
12 teaspoons baking powder
2 teaspoons vanilla
10 cups flour (or as much as needed to spoon cookies out onto cookie sheet)

Preheat oven to 350°F. Combine all ingredients. Spoon out onto cookie sheets. Bake 10–15 minutes.

Cousin June's Anise Cookies

Cousin June baked these cookies every holiday. They were then lovingly mailed to Vietnam, New Jersey, Florida, or wherever her children were at the time. I remember eating one of these cookies still warm from the oven, watching Uncle Lenny dunking one in his coffee. These cookies get better tasting the harder they get.

6 eggs
7 cups flour
2 cups sugar
7 teaspoons baking power
1½ cups Crisco
1 cup milk
1 bottle of anise favoring
1 teaspoon vanilla flavoring

Preheat oven to 350°F. Mix together flour, sugar, and baking powder. Cut in the Crisco as if you were making pie dough. Add milk, eggs, anise, and vanilla.

Grease a cookie sheet. Make a loaf about 5 inches wide and 1½ inches high (I have better luck making two loaves).

Bake until golden brown. Remove from the oven and cut into ¾-inch slices and place sideways on cookie sheets. Brush with a little beaten egg (for a shiny top) and place under the broiler, browning the first side for 10 minutes. Turn, brush with egg again, and brown the other side for 10 minutes.

Pasticiotti

This is my specialty. It's a small pie with pudding inside. My father's first cousin, Frances Paone, from Canastota, taught me how to make "pastis" and it has become my signature dessert. My son-in-law loves them! The cream melts in your mouth and the crust is like a soft yummy cookie.

CRUST

   4 cups flour
   2 eggs
   1 cup sugar
   1 teaspoon vanilla
   2 teaspoon baking powder
   ½ cup milk
   1 cup Crisco

CREAM FILLING (PUDDING)

   ½ cup sugar
   3 tablespoons cornstarch
   2 egg yolks
   2 cups milk

Pinch salt
¼ teaspoon vanilla
Dot butter
Lemon rind

Preheat oven to 325°F. Combine dry ingredients, cut in Crisco, and add vanilla, eggs, milk, and mix well. Carefully roll out the crust (it will be very moist). Cut circles with cookie cutters to fit your tins. I use the big red plastic cups that soda comes in at fast-food places. It's the perfect size. Blend the filling ingredients well and cook in a pan over medium-high heat until thickened.

For chocolate: Omit lemon and add cocoa.

Grease tins well, line tart tins with dough, fill with cream, top with dough, and brush with egg white. Bake, watching carefully, until just golden brown.

Ricotta Pie
(Italian Easter Pie)

Each year, my Great Aunt Jenny (Vencenza Count) made this pie at Easter time. She taught me how to make it during one of my many visits to the JanRicky Camp on Canadarago Lake, just north of Cooperstown. Italian Easter Pie or Ricotta Pie is filled with good things from the kitchen. She said you must have a piece of this pie at Easter to keep you healthy all year long. My Aunt passed away many years ago, so now I make ten of these pies each year at Easter. I make sure everyone I love has a piece. It's just not Easter without it. I think of Uncle Carl and Aunt Jenny every time I make it. They were two lovely souls who had no other motives but to love their family and enjoy life to the fullest.

CRUST
   ¼ cup shortening
   ¼ cup less 1 teaspoon sugar
   1 small egg
   1 teaspoon baking powder
   ¼ cup milk
   1¼ cups less 1 teaspoon flour
FILLING
   1 lb. Ricotta cheese
   ⅔ cup Sugar
   ⅓ teaspoon cinnamon
   1 small Hershey's Almond Bar, broken into bits
   Orange rind/juice
   6 eggs
   ⅓ can evaporated milk
   ¼ container less 1 teaspoon Certo

Preheat oven to 350°F. Mix shortening, sugar, egg, baking powder, milk, and flour to make crust. Press into pie pan. Mix filling ingredients together and pour into crust. Bake for 1 hour or until your knife can cut into the center and come out clean. Let it cool. Sprinkle with confectioner's sugar and serve.

Cousin Carla's Cranberry Pistachio Biscotti

Cousin Carla never goes anywhere empty-handed. Along with her endless smile, she brings homemade baked goods. It's a joy to have her come visit. She and I get together at least once a month for a meal or at least a cup of tea and something she baked.

   2¼ cups all-purpose flour
   1½ teaspoons baking powder
   ½ teaspoon salt

6 tablespoons unsalted butter,
   at room temperature
¾ cup sugar
2 eggs
1 teaspoon lemon juice
1½ teaspoons vanilla extract
½ teaspoon anise flavoring
1 cup dried sweetened cranberries
¾ cup pistachios, shelled

Preheat oven to 325°F. Line a large baking sheet with parchment paper. Sift together the flour, baking powder, and salt, and set aside.

In a large bowl, blend the butter and sugar with an electric mixer. Add and beat in the lemon juice, vanilla, and anise. Add the flour mixture and stir until just blended. Add the cranberries and pistachios. The dough will be sticky.

Turn dough onto a lightly floured surface. Knead 5–6 times using a little flour to make the dough manageable. Divide in half. Shape each half into a rectangle approximately 11″ × 3½″. Carefully transfer to a baking sheet. Bake until just lightly browned, 28–32 minutes. Cool on the baking sheet for 10 minutes.

The biscotti will "finish baking" as it cools, resulting in a soft biscotti. If you prefer a harder biscotti, bake a bit longer. When cool, cut diagonally into 1-inch slices. Yields approximately 20.

Angela Conte's Italian Chocolate Cookies

My mother made these around the holidays, and after I had my own place I started making them. I don't remember a Christmas or Thanksgiving without these cookies.

4 cups flour
1 cup Crisco
1 cup sugar
2 cups warm milk
1 cup cocoa
2 teaspoons baking powder
½ teaspoon baking soda
½ teaspoon nutmeg
½ teaspoon cloves
1 teaspoon cinnamon
1 teaspoon black pepper

Preheat oven to 350°F. Pretty simple: Mix, chill, drop, bake. Mix it well. I normally do all the dry ingredients first, and then add the Crisco, dripping warm milk over it to help soften it. Mix well, then stick it in the fridge. Once it's cooled, roll into little balls and bake. I coat these with a glaze. You can add nuts, raisins, or chocolate chips if you want.

Bake 8–10 minutes, being careful not to let them burn. Cookies should be soft but not chewy.

Almond Cookies

1 cup flour
½ cup butter or margarine, softened
½ cup almonds, crushed
1 teaspoon almond extract
¼ teaspoon salt
¼ cup confectioner's sugar

Preheat oven to 325°F. In a large bowl, mix all ingredients. Take a teaspoon of dough and shape it like a crescent. You don't have to, but they look nice that way. Sometimes I just make them round. Place on a cookie sheet, 1 inch apart. Bake about 20 minutes or until lightly golden. Smells so good.

Almond Macaroons

8 ounce can almond paste
1 cup sugar
2 large egg whites
Red candied cherries
Whole almonds

Preheat oven to 350°F. In a large bowl, mix the almond paste and sugar until smooth. Add egg whites and beat until smooth. Form little balls and press an almond or a cherry into each one. Place on a parchment-lined pan and bake at 18–20 minutes or until lightly browned. These are a must at every holiday, birthday, graduation—you name it.

Farfellette
(Aunt Frances's Fried Bow Cookies)

Okay, I've never made these, but I've eaten my fair share.

2 eggs
2 tablespoons sugar
2 cups flour
2 tablespoons vanilla
1 teaspoon grated lemon zest
Oil for frying
Confectioner's sugar

Beat the eggs and sugar. Stir in 1½ cups of flour, vanilla, and lemon zest. Shape into a ball and knead until smooth. Divide the dough into 4 parts and place under a towel to keep from drying out. Roll each part to ⅛ of an inch think. Cut into about 5 1½-inch strips with a pastry wheel. (Aunt Fran had a cutter with a ruffled edge that made them come out nice and pretty.) Make a slit in the center of each strip. Now take one end and run it through that hole you just made, making a bow. Fry in about 4 inches of hot oil. (Aunt Frances said to take a cube of white bread and drop it in the oil. If it turns golden brown in 50 seconds, the oil is perfect.) Do 3 or 4 cookies at a time for 3 minutes, turning once. Drain on paper towels or brown paper bags. Sprinkle with confectioners sugar.

Half Moon Cookies

Utica is famous for Half Moon Cookies. This is a recipe we've been using for years.

COOKIES
    1½ cups sugar
    ½ cup shortening
    2 eggs
    3½ cups flour
    2 tablespoons baking powder
    1 teaspoon salt
    1 tablespoon pure vanilla
    1 cup milk
FROSTING
    2 cups confectioners sugar
    1 teaspoon of vanilla
    Milk
    2 tablespoons butter
    ¼ cup dried cocoa powder

Preheat oven to 375°F. Mix all the cookie ingredients in a bowl until batter is fluffy and mixed well.

Drop by heaping tablespoons on a greased cookie sheet, making sure they're uniformly round. (I use parchment paper instead of a greased pan.) Bake until lightly browned. Cool completely.

For the white frosting, combine half the sugar, half the vanilla, and add milk a tablespoon at a time until desired thickness to spread. Add one tablespoon softened butter. Frost half of each cookie on the flat side (not the rounded side).

For the chocolate frosting, combine the remaining sugar and vanilla, and again add milk a little at a time until thick enough. Add the remaining butter and cocoa and mix until smooth and frost the other sides of the cookies. (You can use canned frosting, but don't tell anyone!)

Cuccidati
(Fig Cookies)

1 pound dried figs, cut into bits
1 pound raisins, cut into bits
½ cup honey
1 cup walnuts, crushed
Zest of 1 lemon
Zest of 1 orange
1 cup chopped hard chocolate, crushed
½ cup apple juice

Preheat oven to 325°F. Crush the nuts and chocolate until fine. Mix with the apple juice and stir well. It should be sort of medium moist. If not, you need to add more juice. My aunt used a meat grinder to get it all chopped up really well. I don't have a meat grinder, so I put it in my food processor. It works!

Prepare dough using any good pie crust recipe.

My aunt told me to flatten out the dough and cut into strips about 2 × 4 inches. Put 1 tablespoon filling in each piece and fold it over (I lay it out flat, spread the filling on it, roll it up like a jelly roll, and slice it). Bake for 20 minutes. Cool and frost.

Frances Paone's Italian White Cookies

My cousin Jeanette gave me this, her mother's recipe, and said she can't think of a nicer way to remember and honor her mother's love for cooking than having it included in this book.

COOKIES
> 6 tablespoons shortening
> 1 cup sugar
> 3 eggs
> ¼ cup milk
> 1 tablespoon vanilla or lemon flavoring
> 4 cups flour
> 6 teaspoons baking powder

FROSTING
> ½ box confectioner's sugar
> 1 teaspoon butter
> 1 tablespoon lemon flavoring
> Milk as needed to make a smooth frosting.

Preheat oven to 375° F. Mix together dry ingredients. Add to wet ingredients. Form small balls and place on a baking sheet. Bake for 10 minutes. Set aside to cool.

Combine frosting ingredients and beat with a mixer.

Vonnie's Kitchen Tips

Sticky Caps
You know how honey and syrup bottles get all sticky under the cap? Here is how to keep that from happening. Before you use the honey or syrup, wipe the threads of the bottle with a little bit of oil. That lid will never stick—it's like a miracle.

To Soften Butter
I never remember to take the butter out of the fridge when I'm baking. Then it's hard as a rock and I try microwaving it and it turns into liquid, forcing me to make popcorn to use it up. Here's a great remedy. Put the stick of butter in a plastic zip lock bag and roll it flat with a rolling pin. It softens up in a few minutes.

Sticky Pasta
Whenever you are making a pasta dish, keep some of the water you cooked the pasta in and use a few spoonfuls if you need it to adjust your sauce thickness.

Pasta Sauce Too Thin?
If you are out of tomato paste and your sauce is a bit too thin, add some Italian bread crumbs.

Herbs and Oils
These are my favorites.
   Olio d'oliva extravergine is extra-virgin olive oil. I only use one brand: Filippo Berio. It's what I'm used to. My mom and dad used it. I am never without a gallon of it in my home and I use it every day.
   Aglio is garlic. Garlic is essential. It has a strong scent and pungent flavor, and can be used in salads, meats, sauces, vegetables, and just about anything else. Amounts

depend on how much you like it. Start out with small amounts and adjust it to your taste.

Basilico is basil. Really, I can't cook without basil. It has a delicate flavor and is mildly fragrant. I always have fresh basil growing in my kitchen, ready to use. You can flavor soups, stews, vegetables, chicken, meat, and sauces with it. And if you ever make a salad without fresh basil, I refuse to eat in your home.

Prezzemolo is parsley. Fresh parsley can be grown anywhere. You then tie it and hang it upside down in the kitchen and you've always got full flavor to add to soups, stews, and fish dishes.

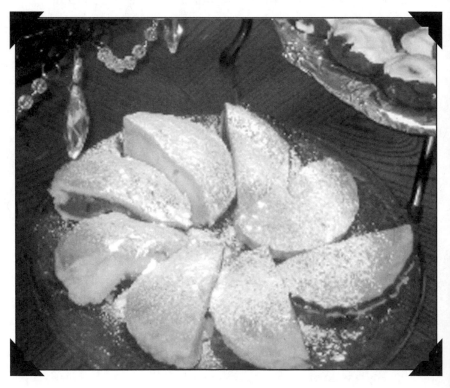

My pasticiotti—and those are Mom's Italian Chocolate
Cookies in the upper righthand corner

Invitation

Please email Yvonne at smile@yvonneconte.com and ask to be put on our free mailing list. You will receive a monthly newsletter with ideas of ways to add joy to your life, communicate better with others, and cope with stress and life's difficulties. Each month, Yvonne tells you where she will be speaking, so you may join her if she is in your neighborhood. Also, you will find quotes and stories from Humor Advantage clients and friends on how they have used humor in their lives. And we would never even think about giving anyone your contact information. We just think that's rude.

Join Humor Advantage on Facebook.
We would love to have you.

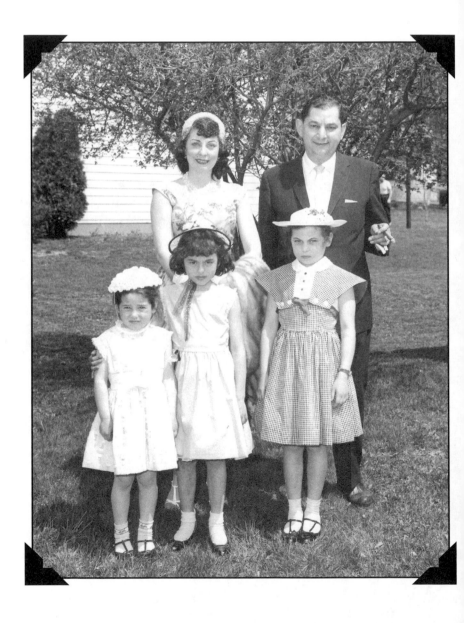

About the Author

Yvonne Conte has been teaching the benefits of Laughter, Humor, and Joy since 1995. She travels extensively as a keynote speaker for conferences, and selectively mentors young speakers with the same passion for making this world a better place for all.

Yvonne's daughter, Aubry Ludington, is married to Todd Panek and they have three handsome boys, Christian, Joey, and Jack, not to mention Princess Leia, the family dog. They live just one mile from Yvonne in Upstate New York. Aubry is a respected workshop facilitator and keynote speaker. Todd is a manager in the insurance industry. Yvonne's son, John Ludington, lives in Northern California with his partner, Andrea, and her daughter Kahvi. John is an accomplished musician and Andrea runs an online boutique.

To contact the author write:
Humor Advantage, Incorporated
4736 Onondaga Blvd., Suite 231
Syracuse, NY 13219
(315) 487-3771
www.yvonneconte.com

FAMILY DISCLAIMER: *The stories in this book come from my memories. Keep in mind that we all recall things differently. Some family members may remember things slightly differently than I do and that's okay. I don't want to give anyone agita. Have a club soda and relax! This is the way I remember it.*